CONCISE GUIDE TO
Ethics in Mental Health Care

Laura Weiss Roberts, M.D.

Professor and Chair
Department of Psychiatry and Behavioral Medicine
Medical College of Wisconsin
Milwaukee, Wisconsin

Allen R. Dyer, M.D., Ph.D.

Professor
Department of Psychiatry and Behavioral Sciences
James H. Quillen College of Medicine
East Tennessee State University
Johnson City, Tennessee

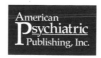

American Psychiatric Publishing, Inc.

Washington, DC
London, England

Copyright © 2004 American Psychiatric Publishing, Inc.
ALL RIGHTS RESERVED

Typeset in Adobe Times and Helvetica

Manufactured in the United States of America on acid-free paper
08 07 06 05 04   5 4 3 2 1
First Edition

American Psychiatric Publishing, Inc.
1000 Wilson Boulevard
Arlington, VA 22209-3901
www.appi.org

Library of Congress Cataloging-in-Publication Data
Roberts, Laura Weiss, 1960-
    Concise guide to ethics in mental health care / Laura Weiss Roberts, Allen R. Dyer.—1st ed.
        p. ; cm. — (Concise guides)
    Includes bibliographical references and index.
    ISBN 0-88048-944-8 (alk. paper)
    1. Psychotherapy—Moral and ethical aspects—Handbooks, manuals, etc. 2. Psychiatric ethics—Handbooks, manuals, etc. I. Dyer, Allen R. II. Title.
    [DNLM: 1. Psychotherapy—Moral and ethical aspects—Handbooks. WM 34 R645c 2003]
RC455.2.E8R63 2003
174.2—dc21   2003056060

British Library Cataloguing-in-Publication Data
A CIP record is available from the British Library.

CONCISE GUIDE TO
Ethics in Mental Health Care

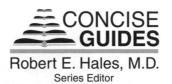

CONCISE
GUIDES

Robert E. Hales, M.D.
Series Editor

CONTENTS

11 Caring for People at End of Life 185

12 Ethical Issues in Psychiatric Genetics
(with Cynthia M. A. Geppert, M.D., Ph.D.) 207

17 Health Care Ethics Committees
(with Tom Townsend, M.D.) 295

LIST OF TABLES

LIST OF FIGURES

CONTRIBUTORS

Jerald Belltz, Ph.D.
Associate Professor, Department of Psychiatry, University of New Mexico Health Sciences Center, Albuquerque, New Mexico

Michael Bogenschutz, M.D.
Associate Professor and Vice Chair, Department of Psychiatry, University of New Mexico Health Sciences Center, Albuquerque, New Mexico

Cynthia M. A. Geppert, M.D., Ph.D.
Assistant Professor, Department of Psychiatry, University of New Mexico Health Sciences Center, Albuquerque, New Mexico

Merry N. Miller, M.D.
Professor and Chair, Department of Psychiatry and Behavioral Sciences, James H. Quillen College of Medicine, East Tennessee State University, Johnson City, Tennessee

Tom Townsend, M.D.
Director, Program in Clinical Ethics, East Tennessee State University, Bristol, Tennessee

INTRODUCTION

to the Concise Guides Series

The Concise Guides Series from American Psychiatric Publishing, Inc., provides, in an accessible format, practical information for psychiatrists, psychiatry residents, and medical students working in a variety of treatment settings, such as inpatient psychiatry units, outpatient clinics, consultation-liaison services, and private office settings. The Concise Guides are meant to complement the more detailed information to be found in lengthier psychiatry texts.

The Concise Guides address topics of special concern to psychiatrists, mental health professionals, and trainees in clinical practice. The books in this series contain a detailed table of contents, along with an index, tables, figures, and other charts for easy access. The books are designed to fit into a lab coat pocket or jacket pocket, which makes them a convenient source of information. References have been limited to those most relevant to the material presented.

Robert E. Hales, M.D., M.B.A.
Series Editor, Concise Guides

PREFACE

Providing ethical care is the aspiration of every dedicated clinician and clinical trainee, and yet fulfilling this ideal is not a simple matter of being—or trying to be—good. Each new day brings encounters with people with serious illnesses whose care is accompanied by new ethical questions and challenges. Each new clinical practice approach, each new technological development, each new cost-containment scheme, and each new social policy creates complex, seemingly unprecedented, and irresolvable dilemmas. Traditions, codes, and legal rulings may provide little help and less comfort in these situations—situations that define the real meaning of professionalism in the care of human suffering.

This book is about approaching the ethical aspects of mental health care—both subtle and dramatic—with clarity, coherence, and optimism. It emphasizes real experience as opposed to disembodied theories, which may cause harm when they are misapplied or are not attuned to clinical realities. As a result, this text does not offer simple answers. Rather, it seeks to provide guideposts, to impart information, to foster skill development, and to encourage openness, collaboration, and self-reflection. These elements, together with tenacious endeavors to be—and to try to be—good, represent a compass and a set of map-making tools for those traveling with their patients along the ethical frontier of mental illness.

■ INTRODUCTION TO THIS BOOK

This Concise Guide encompasses fundamental ethics principles and skills and addresses topics of special importance in mental health care, such as the ethical use of power in high-risk situations, informed consent, and confidentiality. It covers special or distinct populations (e.g., children, clinicians) and particular contexts for care (e.g., small communities, managed care settings). Each chapter contains case examples that may be used in independent study or in small-group discussions. At the back of the book, we have included a glossary of ethics terms and a list of additional resource materials.

■ ACKNOWLEDGMENTS

The authors wish to thank Dr. Cynthia Geppert for her valuable and tireless efforts in the development of this book. We also offer our appreciation and acknowledgment for the authors who contributed to this book: Dr. Jerald Belitz, Dr. Michael Bogenschutz, Dr. Merry Miller, and Dr. Tom Townsend.

Dr. Roberts expresses her appreciation and gratitude to her colleague, coauthor, and new friend, Dr. Dyer, whose collegiality and kindness are unparalleled. She also wishes to express her love and thanks to her husband, Brian; her children, Madeline, Helen, Willa, and Tommy; her mom, Anne; and her friends, Rosalina and Teresita, for their generosity of spirit in all things but especially their patience during the writing of this text. She also extends her appreciation to colleagues, Dr. Sally Severino, Dr. Joel Yager, Ms. Megan Smithpeter, and Ms. Kristin Edenharder, for their encouragement and many contributions to this work.

Dr. Dyer would like to thank Dr. Roberts for the invitation to work on this project, which proved to be both rewarding and fun, and the contributing authors, who offered such thoughtful commentary and discussion. He would also like to express his love and appreciation to his wife, Sue, for her support over three and a half decades, and to their sons, Will and Cliff, who now carry ethical reflection into their own careers.

ETHICS: PRINCIPLES AND PROFESSIONALISM

Ethics refers to ways of understanding and examining moral life to create a coherent sense of what is good and right in human experience. Ethics is an endeavor that requires sensitivity, knowledge, and skill. It is informed by scholarship and evidence and shaped by values and context. It is a branch of philosophy insofar as philosophy is the discipline involving rational thinking, but ethics is not just about thinking. It is also about feeling, observing, experiencing, and right action, and these involve all of life. In health care, the study of ethics has helped to develop principles and decision-making approaches that guide clinical practice. It also has helped to clarify how the health professions can best fulfill their responsibilities in serving patients, communities, and society.

Ethics in mental health care is exceptionally complex, in part because of the nature of mental illnesses—which, by definition, affect an individual's most fundamental human capacities, relationships, and social roles. Mental illnesses affect aspects of life that we define as fundamental to being human, such as perceptions, feelings, relatedness, self-understanding, and choices. In addition, people who struggle with mental illness may be isolated, misunderstood, and stigmatized and have few resources to overcome barriers in their lives, including limited access to appropriate care. Moreover, the treatment of mental illness involves techniques that require exploration of intimate aspects of patients' lives and interventions that in some cases may limit the freedoms of patients who are at risk of harming themselves or others. People with mental illness may have exceptional strengths, but they also may have exceptional vulnerabilities. Ensuring the ethical use of the power entrusted to clinicians in these situations is very challenging. For these reasons, ethics lies at the very heart of mental health care.

Skills that clinicians working in mental health care can bring to ethics are many. For example, astute clinical care in this area requires an attentiveness to the importance of human experience in relation to illness and suffering. Beyond eliciting symptoms, recognizing patterns, and treating disease, mental health care involves attention to the experience of losing one's sense of being healthy and whole that accompanies a major depressive episode, the experience of perceiving voices that others do not hear in living with schizophrenia, the experience of surviving an event that forever changes one's views of oneself and the world in posttraumatic stress disorder, and the experience of feeling one's insight and abilities slip away in chronic progressive illnesses. Gaining an understanding of how these experiences intersect with the strengths, vulnerabilities, choices, hopes, development, and life history of the individual is essential to good clinical care. Awareness of such aspects of the illness experience requires sensitivity, attunement, and integration of diverse, dynamic influences, ranging from biological deficits to personal values. Paying attention to these elements of a patient's care prepares one well for clarifying and addressing complex ethical considerations in the patient's care.

A second skill that clinicians working in mental health bring to ethics is a commitment to understanding how one's own motivations, attitudes, values, life history, and behaviors may influence therapeutic interactions with patients. These insights bring with them a professional commitment to honest self-observation and to the habit of tracking one's own internal responses to patients to discern biases and gaps in judgment. These "habits" of sound clinical practice in mental health care are extraordinarily important to ethical reflection and decision making as well.

A third, closely related skill is the recognition that excellence in one's work and continuing efforts to improve one's skills are the first duty of the clinician in this field. Beyond this, however, the role in which one serves often shapes the nature and limits of one's professional obligations. For example, mental health clinicians function in a variety of roles, ranging from forensic consultant to school-based caregiver, from emergency room clinician to psychotherapist, from psychopharmacological subspecialist to case manager. These roles carry with them diverse duties and, at times, divided loyalties. The psychologist performing "fitness for duty" evaluations of active-duty military personnel must share his or her findings with the commanding officer; a case manager may need to report suspected child neglect or parole violation after a home visit. Given the significant, sensitive character of these activities in the realm of mental health, awareness of the special ethical commitments of each kind of role is particularly important for this field.

Other gifts that mental health clinicians bring to ethics include attentiveness to processes of human interaction and awareness of the contribution of conflict and unconscious elements in individual, interpersonal, and group interactions. Clinicians working with people with mental illness will also recognize that there is more to ethics than rational thought. Unconscious motives, feelings, drives, and conflicts—both internal (indecision or guilt) and external (from argument to warfare)—both inform and are informed by ethics. Ethics is born in conflict, and to be useful it must offer help in resolving the conflicts that are central to human existence. Mental health clinicians furthermore are accustomed to working with colleagues of different backgrounds and disciplines in the course of providing care to patients, and this interdependence is a valuable approach to identifying and resolving ethical problems that may be overlooked when one practices in isolation.

In this chapter, we describe the principles of traditional ethics as they have emerged and evolved within the clinical professions.

■ TRADITIONAL PRINCIPLES OF THE CLINICAL PROFESSIONS

Historically, medicine as a healing art traces its ethical foundations to the writings of Hippocrates, who lived in Greece 25 centuries ago. Hippocrates is considered the father of modern medicine because his approach was scientific—in that he tried to observe systematically the course of illnesses—yet he stood as a priest in the religious or shamanistic tradition. Hippocrates was both a naturalist and a spiritual healer. He taught a loyal family of "student-sons" under a plane tree on the island of Kos. Remains of a temple at which he practiced can be visited today. It was laid out on three levels, with columned sanctuaries on the highest level, containing defined niches for all of the gods and goddesses of the pantheon, available for supplication, and barracks, or pavilions, in which patients could reside near the mineral springs, positioned with views of the blue-green waters of the Aegean Sea, where warm sea breezes ventilated the most comfortable temperatures. Add a healthful diet and the attentive care of Hippocrates' family, and all the ingredients for healing were present. Confucian writings from around the same period speak of similar virtues: humanness, compassion, and filial piety. The writings of Maimonides and those from the various religious traditions more than 2,000 years ago likewise offer much inspiration, some guidance, and special demands for adherence to healers in all generations.

These concepts underlying the ethics of healing have been reclaimed by modern physicians and other health professions: a band of healers, united by a shared commitment to articulated principles of ethics. Of the key principles of the Hippocratic tradition (Table 1–1), the most prominent is *beneficence*—the use of one's expertise exclusively to help the ill: "I will act only for the benefit of the patient." Closely linked to beneficence is the memorable Hippocratic aphorism, "First, do no harm." The fact that the phrase is given to us in Latin, *Primum non nocere,* probably stems from 19th and early 20th century British and American physicians, who studied Latin, used a Latin vocabulary for much of medicine, and wrote prescriptions in Latin. This early commitment to ethical principles gave medicine a touch of both mysticism and erudition, establishing the dual tradition so cherished by healers and sick alike: medicine can be viewed as both religious and scientific, as an art and as a science. These principles offer a useful point of departure for considering the dilemmas and conflicts that have emerged with the new technologies of modern medicine.

TABLE 1–1.	Ethical principles articulated in the Hippocratic writings

Beneficence ("I will come for the benefit of the sick")

Confidentiality ("What I see in the lives of men, I will not noise abroad")

Proscription against sex with patients (mischief, exploitation of vulnerability)

Proscription against euthanasia ("I will not give a deadly drug, nor suggest such a thing")

Proscription against abortion ("I will not give a woman an abortive remedy")

Practice within the limits of competence (I will not "cut on the stone")

Hope and optimism (*On Decorum* suggests not offering a "gloomy" prognosis)

Nonmaleficence (neologism for "first, do no harm")

Professional affiliations (associate only with those who have sworn by *The Oath*)

■ PROFESSIONALISM AND THE EVOLUTION OF BIOETHICAL PRINCIPLES

A profession is entrusted with fulfilling special responsibilities in society. Medicine involves the use of specialized expertise and wisdom to enhance and preserve the lives of others, seeking to foster their health and well-being, to diminish their suffering, and to do so with honor, compassion, and respect. Six principles in particular have been identified as encompassing the basic ethical values on which complex, ethically important decisions may be made by health professionals: beneficence, autonomy, nonmaleficence, justice, veracity, and fidelity (Beauchamp and Childress 2001). The tensions and shifting emphases among these principles reveal much about social change and the place of medicine, especially during recent decades, in which technological developments have been extraordinary. They also set the stage for issues that health care, ethics, and society must address in the years ahead.

Beneficence, the duty to "do good," is intrinsically the subject matter of ethics. What does it mean to do good? From the standpoint of the moral agent, one who is motivated to do good, it means to do right by others. For physicians since antiquity, beneficence has implied doing right by patients, a duty understood as a question for physicians to determine, although healers could hardly remain oblivious to the needs of those they cared for. Beneficence could not and cannot be understood apart from its relationship with a corollary principle: respect for autonomy.

Autonomy, which can be understood simply as self-determination, is based in the fundamental imperative of *respect for persons.* It is linked with the concept of *privacy,* which in our society is understood as the right to have one's body or mind not be intruded upon. It is also linked with the concept of *voluntarism,* which encompasses the ability to act in accordance with one's authentic sense of what is good, right, and best in light of one's situation, values, and prior history. Voluntarism further entails the capacity to make this choice freely and in the absence of coercion. In this construction, beneficence is thus to be judged by the recipient, not just by the initiator. In legal terms, we now understand and accept that patients have a right to self-determination; thus, everything that a physician does must be done with the consent of the patient. Beneficence untempered by autonomy was often paternalistic, relying inordinately on the wisdom and conscience of the physician without sufficient regard for the perspective and values of the patient.

As medical technology came to offer more options for care and as society became more rights-oriented, patients increasingly began to claim more authority in the process of making medical decisions (in the 1970s and 1980s). There was a gradual and perceptible shift from beneficence as the keystone of medical ethics to autonomy as the dominant principle of bioethics. Although this shift gave patients a larger hand in medical decision making, physicians still saw patients who asked to be told what to do or what to choose. Autonomy also carried with it the idea that because patients made the choices, physicians' sole role was to offer the technology (Churchill 1995). Autonomy could degenerate into indifference or a materialistic commercialism. Many physicians understand that beneficence carried with it affirmative obligations. Psychiatrists and mental health professionals understand autonomy as an ideal, not a presupposition. Self-determination is an achievement, even a goal, of both physical and psychotherapeutic treatment.

Nonmaleficence is a new word coined in the 1970s to express the principle behind the oft-quoted aphorism, "First, do no harm." "Harm" is a key consideration in therapeutic interventions that may result in adverse effects or outcomes—for example, medication for psychosis can cause tardive dyskinesia or increase the risk of bone marrow suppression or of developing diabetes. The principle of nonmaleficence is also critical in research, a venue that is dedicated not solely to patient benefit but also to a scientific task and that involves a calculation of risk versus benefit.

The principle of justice brings equitable distribution of power and resources into ethical focus. On an individual level, the tensions between beneficence and autonomy assume a locus of decision making somewhere between the physician and patient. On a societal level, distributive-justice questions arise in regard to fair allocation of resources. What access to care, expertise, and other health resources might an individual patient reasonably expect in a just society? What obligations do a physician or health care provider owe a particular patient, and what roles can providers play in providing or limiting resources to particular individuals? How do providers understand their obligations to society as well as to those they serve directly? These questions might once have been perceived as beyond the scope of medicine and of health care, understood either in technical or humanistic terms. Their resolution depends on an understanding of what constitutes a just society and the respective roles of the citizens, including clinicians, who play a direct role in allocation decisions. The major tensions in these debates center on concepts of social justice. Libertarian views hold that the highest political ideal is freedom; socialist views hold that equality is the highest distributive ideal. More practically nuanced views of justice derive from Immanuel Kant's views of welfare justice as elaborated by John Rawls, which hold that the ideal state is founded on a contract in which its members have the freedom to seek happiness up to the point that one person's pursuit of happiness does not limit another person's freedom to pursue happiness (Sterba 1995). Although these considerations seem abstract, their applications are quite practical.

The move from beneficence to autonomy as a dominant ethical principle was accompanied by a shift of the locus of decision making from the doctor to the patient, or more broadly from professional to client—the very term *client* suggesting a self-determining agent. The move to justice, seen in economic terms, removed the locus of decision making from the doctor and the patient (now considered "providers" and "consumers"). The consequence of this shift for health care professionals was that economic aspects of care began to intrude and to demand attention in ways that seemed novel and perplexing. Ethical principles must be understood within their social and economic contexts and cannot be separated from considerations of justice, which go beyond the doctor–patient (or professional–client) relationships.

Veracity is the principle of telling the truth. It is a positive duty to express the truth, but it also involves the obligation to not deceive through omission. *Fidelity* is the principle of serving faithfully—and often exclusively—a person or an explicit positive aim. These two principles have become very important in recent years in relation to conflicting roles and conflicts of interest. For example, disclosure (i.e., telling the truth) has become a primary safeguard surrounding conflicts of interest in clinical practice and human investigation, which can pose threats to exclusively serving the well-being of patients and research participants.

Modern formulations of these principles are being proposed and considered. The cardinal elements of the Professionalism Charter consensus document are listed in Table 1–2. In addition, Davidoff (2000) proposed seven key ethical principles for health care professionals:

1. Rights—People have a right to health and health care.
2. Balance—Care of individual patients is central, but the health of populations is also our concern.
3. Comprehensiveness—In addition to treating illness, we have an obligation to ease suffering, minimize disability, prevent disease, and promote health.

4. Cooperation—Health care succeeds only if we cooperate with those we serve, each other, and those in other sectors.
5. Improvement—Improving health care is a serious and continuing responsibility.
6. Safety—Do no harm.
7. Openness—Being open, honest, and trustworthy is vital in health care.

TABLE 1–2.   **Charter on medical professionalism**

Preamble

Professionalism is the basis of medicine's contract with society. It demands placing the interests of patients above those of the physician, setting and maintaining standards of competence and integrity, and providing expert advice to society on matters of health. The principles and responsibilities of medical professionalism must be clearly understood by both the profession and society. Essential to this contract is public trust in physicians, which depends on the integrity of both individual physicians and the whole profession.

Fundamental principles

Principle of primacy of patient welfare
Principle of patient autonomy
Principle of social justice

A set of professional responsibilities

Commitment to professional competence
Commitment to honesty with patients
Commitment to patient confidentiality
Commitment to maintaining appropriate relations with patients
Commitment to improving quality of care
Commitment to improving access to care
Commitment to a just distribution of finite resources
Commitment to scientific knowledge
Commitment to maintaining trust by managing conflicts of interest
Commitment to professional responsibilities

Source.   Developed and advanced by the American Board of Internal Medicine Foundation, the American College of Physicians–American Society of Internal Medicine, and the European Federation of Internal Medicine. Full text is available at: http://www.annals.org/issues/v136n3/full/200202050-00012.html#top.

■ PRINCIPLES, RULES, AND CONTEXTUALISM

Principles differ from rules. Principle-based ethics are also called *teleological* ethics, from the Greek *telos,* meaning "end" or "goal," and rule-based ethics are also called *deontological* ethics (Frankena 1963). Teleological ethics emphasizes outcomes and intent toward those outcomes, whereas deontological ethics emphasizes prior imperatives as determining choices in ethical dilemmas. In outlining a list of principles that the conscientious practitioner might wish to follow, we recognize that those principles require application and that application is subject to ambiguity—and, indeed, self-deception and even corruption. On the other hand, rules (legal rules in particular) carry the force of civil law; religious rules carry whatever sanctions one holds sacred. Thus, in United States law, the Constitution is the ultimate deontological arbiter as determined by the Supreme Court, and the Ten Commandments is perhaps the best example of a deontological ethic, "cast in stone" and (relatively) unambiguous: "Thou shalt not kill." Deontological ethics offers a clarity and a certain security, but even such a seemingly unambiguous commandment has certain exceptions: the just war, the conflict between one life and another, the types of dilemmas that physicians may encounter. In sum, the realities of medical situations inspire teleological thinking among even the most committed deontologists.

Clinical situations thus make contextualists out of all conscientious professionals. *Contextualism* is a form of teleology that holds that the rightness of a particular decision depends on the context. In ethical reflection, contextualism accepts the argument "It all depends..." but demands an explication of how the context or situation might affect the decision. The introduction of material economic considerations into clinical decisions is an example of such contextualism. Clinicians rightly feel torn between their felt obligations to their patients or clients and their obligations to society and its economic resources. They have divided loyalties and divided duties, and they may not be able to escape an ethical bind.

The form of ethical analysis that examines the situation and all relevant principles, rules, history, and meaning is referred to as *casuistry.* Casuistry is similar to the law in this respect, although the aim is to discern not what one *can or must* do in order to comply with shared rules of the community or society, but rather what one *may or, at times, ought to choose,* given the situation at hand. Other valuable approaches, such as virtue-based ethics, which emphasizes the qualities of the moral agent evaluating and enacting a choice, are summarized in Table 1–3. A full analysis of these approaches is beyond the scope of this book; readings for the interested professional are provided in Appendix B at the end of this book. It is important to note, however, that clinicians tend to be eclectic, dynamic, and pragmatic, employing valuable elements of each of these approaches. In Chapter 2, we outline a clinical ethics decision-making strategy and key ethics skills for professionals working with mentally ill individuals. In addition, the ethical traditions of professions are symbolized by ethical codes such as the Hippocratic Oath and the Declaration of Geneva (professional codes and guidelines are discussed in greater detail in Chapter 17). These codes and guidelines function not deontologically as a list of rules, but more fundamentally in a teleological mode as goals toward which the professional strives (Dyer 1998).

All of these approaches affirm the healing role and special duties of clinicians in caring for the sick and in seeking to promote the health and well-being of individual patients, vulnerable populations, and society broadly. The clinical professions carry the highest ideals: service, duty, honor, commitment to patients, self-sacrifice, and the doing and making of good. In essence, clinical work is not merely an occupation; it is a profession—and for some, perhaps, a vocation—and it is a privilege dedicated to the well-being of others. New conceptions of professionalism reclaim, reaffirm, and perhaps may redefine the ethical underpinnings of healing activity and emphasize the clinician's dual contract to patient and society (Table 1–4).

TABLE 1–3. Models of ethical thinking

Model	Major figure	Key features	Strengths	Limitations
Utilitarianism, or the ethics of consequences	John Stewart Mill	Weigh the consequences of actions and rules. Those that bring about the greatest good for the most people are most ethical.	Useful in formulating public policy because it requires impartial assessment of all interests. Has beneficence as a goal.	Difficult to translate into practice. Immoral practices may be justified. May demand that the minority sacrifice too much for the majority.
Deontology, or the ethics of duty	Immanuel Kant	There is an absolute good and right. To be ethical, persons must fulfill these absolute duties unconditionally.	There are some moral judgments that apply in almost all circumstances to everyone (e.g., respect for persons).	Conflicting obligations. Too much emphasis on law, not enough on relationships. Very abstract.
Casuistry, or case ethics	Albert Jonsen	Taking specific circumstances into account when applying rules, norms and principles to particular cases. Reasons by analogy from similar types of cases.	Emphasizes context and precedent rather than abstract theory. Does not need a principle to make a moral judgment.	Analogies from other types of cases may miss uniqueness of case. Circumstances of case may not lead to resolution without theory.

TABLE 1–3.	Models of ethical thinking *(continued)*			
Model	Major figure	Key features	Strengths	Limitations
Care ethics	Carol Gilligan	Focus on care, responsibility, and trust involved in relationships. Commitment to others rather than individual autonomy is the basis of the ethical life.	Emphasizes relationships and emotions rather than principles and reason. Emphasizes women's experience of ethical life.	Caring may impair objectivity. May neglect necessary principles.
Virtue ethics	Edmund Pellegrino and David Thomasma	Ethical decisions are rooted in qualities or character, such as honesty and faithfulness. Actions are right only if they are what a virtuous person would do in the same situation.	Internal values and habits rather than external rules and imperatives. Highlights importance of motive and character.	Virtue may be too unclear or pluralistic to serve as a basis for judgment. Persons may act wrongly out of virtue (e.g., withhold the truth from a dying patient to avoid upsetting him or her).

TABLE 1–3. Models of ethical thinking *(continued)*

Model	Major figure	Key features	Strengths	Limitations
Principle-based ethics	James Childress and Thomas Beauchamp	General principles and rules are primary in ethical decision making and action. Ethical dilemmas are resolved through the balancing and specification of various principles.	Represents broad moral considerations that can be applied to specific situations. Presents a method of resolving conflicts between ethical principles.	Emphasizes action and reason at the expense of character and emotion. May neglect the experience of women. May be applied mechanically.

Acknowledgment. Cynthia M.A. Geppert, M.D., Ph.D., provided assistance in preparing this table.

TABLE 1–4.   **Definitions of professionalism**

Professionalism is the demonstration in practice of aptitudes, attributes, and attitudes to which practitioners lay claim and which might reasonably be demanded of them by those entrusted to their care, and by their colleagues "of good repute and competency." Its hallmark is commitment: (i) to the individual patient, requiring *professional courtesy,* continuing competence, personal *integrity,* and advocacy of the patient's interests; (ii) to the *health care system,* ensuring continuity of relevant care of the highest possible quality for all without discrimination; and (iii) to the profession, entailing active "allegiance to the bodies providing collective professional responsibility" (Boyd et al. 1997).

Professionals are usually identified by their commitment to provide important services to clients or consumers and by their specialized training. Professions maintain self-regulating organizations that control entry into occupational roles by formally certifying that candidates have acquired the necessary knowledge and skills. The concept of a medical professional is closely tied to a background of distinctive education and skills that patients typically lack and that morally must be used to benefit patients. In learned professions, such as medicine, the background knowledge of the professional derives from closely supervised training, and the professional is one who provides a service to others (Beauchamp and Childress 2001).

Profession…noun…1: the act of taking vows of a religious community; 2: an act of openly declaring or publicly claiming a belief, faith, or opinion: Protestation; 3: an avowed religious faith; 4a: a calling requiring specialized knowledge and often long and intensive academic preparation; 4b: a principal calling, vocation, or employment; 4c: the whole body of persons engaged in a calling (Webster's Tenth Collegiate Dictionary 1994, p. 930).

A profession may be defined in terms of its knowledge, technology, or expertise, or it may be defined in terms of its ethics and values…. A profession that understands itself in terms of its knowledge, technology, or expertise may be bartered in the marketplace (Dyer 1998).

A profession is a socially sanctioned activity whose primary object is the well-being of others above the professional's personal gain (Racy 1990).

TABLE 1–4.   **Definitions of professionalism _(continued)_**

"Being a professional is an ethical matter, entailing devotion to a way of life, in the service of others and of some higher good.... These special considerations imply specific and inherently medical obligations both of omission and commission, as well as appropriately reverential stance of the physician before his chosen profession" (Kass 1983, p. 1305).

Justice Louis Brandeis believed that a profession had three features: training that was intellectual and involved knowledge, as distinguished from skill; work that was pursued primarily for others and not for oneself; and success that was measured by more than the amount of financial return (Brandeis 1993).

A set of values, attitudes, and behaviors that results in serving the interests of patients and society before one's own (Reynolds 1994).

Professionalism is not a matter of _trying_ but of _being_ (LaCombe 1993).

The core of professionalism constitutes "...those attitudes and behaviors that serve to maintain patient interest above physician self-interest. Accordingly, professionalism...aspires to altruism, accountability, excellence, duty, service, honor, integrity, and respect for others" (Stobo and Blank 1994).

■ REFERENCES

Beauchamp TL, Childress JF: Principles of Biomedical Ethics, 5th Edition. New York, Oxford University Press, 2001

Boyd KM, Higgs R, Pinching AJ: The New Dictionary of Medical Ethics. London, BMJ Publishing, 1997

Brandeis LD: Business: A Profession. Boston, MA, Hole, Cushman, & Flint, 1993

Churchill LR: Beneficence, in Encyclopedia of Bioethics, Revised Edition. Edited by Reich WT. New York, Macmillan, 1995, pp 243–247

Davidoff F: Changing the subject: ethical principles for everyone in health care. Ann Intern Med 133:386–389, 2000

Dyer AR: Ethics and Psychiatry: Toward Professional Definition. Washington, DC, American Psychiatric Press, 1998

Frankena WR: Ethics. Englewood Cliffs, NJ, Prentice Hall Professional Technical Reference, 1963

Kass LR: Professing ethically. On the place of ethics in defining medicine. JAMA 249:1305–1310, 1983

LaCombe MA: On professionalism. Am J Med 94:329, 1993

Merriam-Webster's Collegiate Dictionary, 10th Edition. Springfield, MA, Merriam-Webster, 1994

Racy J: Professionalism: sane and insane [editorial]. J Clin Psychiatry 51:138–140, 1990

Reynolds PP: Reaffirming professionalism through the education community [see comments]. Ann Intern Med 120:609–614, 1994

Sterba JP: Justice, in Encyclopedia of Bioethics, Revised Edition. Edited by Reich WT. New York, Macmillan, 1995, pp 1308–1315

Stobo JD, Blank LL: American Board of Internal Medicine's Project Professionalism: staying ahead of the wave. Am J Med 97:1–3, 1994

2

CLINICAL DECISION-MAKING AND ETHICS SKILLS

Clinicians working in the realm of mental health and mental illness are often well prepared to address ethical considerations in caring for people with mental illness. Mental health professionals attend to motivations that underlie choices and behaviors, and they have a sense of the importance of insight, values, psychological development, and personal history in the lives of their patients, as individuals and as moral persons in society. They understand self-observation and self-scrutiny to be essential "habits" in assuring clinical excellence. All of these characteristics help to foster optimal ethical reflection and rigorous decision making in patient care, and it is often these qualities that lead individuals to choose the field of psychiatry.

Beyond these personal qualities, there are several essential ethics skills that should be in the "tool kit" of all clinical professionals working with people with mental illness (Table 2–1). The clinician's repertoire should also include a specific and focused strategy for approaching ethical decisions in clinical care (Morenz and Sales 1997). One such model is described in a step-by-step fashion in this chapter. These skills and intentional decision-making strategy may be used in enacting clinical practices that are ethically important, such as obtaining informed consent and preserving confidentiality, and in caring for special populations, as described throughout this book.

TABLE 2–1.	**Essential ethics skills in clinical practice**

The ability to identify the ethical features of a patient's care

The ability to see how one's own life experiences, attitudes, and knowledge may influence one's care of a patient

The ability to identify one's areas of clinical expertise (i.e., scope of clinical competence) and to work within those boundaries

The ability to anticipate ethically risky or problematic situations

The ability to gather additional information and to seek consultation and additional expertise in order to clarify and, ideally, resolve the conflict

The ability to build additional ethical safeguards into the patient care situation

■ ETHICS SKILLS IN MENTAL HEALTH CARE

The first essential ethical skill is *the ability to identify the ethical features of a patient's care.* This involves sensitivity and an ability to apply ethical principles such as respect for persons, beneficence, autonomy, nonmaleficence, justice, veracity, and fidelity. It involves an up-front appreciation for how the use of an alternative decision maker is different, for example, in arriving at a hospitalization decision for an elderly person with early Alzheimer's disease, an adult with bipolar affective disorder, a young adult with Down syndrome, or a child in need of an appendectomy. In providing mental health care, it is important to discern how the patient's distinct cultural background, religious or spiritual beliefs, and personal history shape the values through which he or she understands the illness process and the decisions he or she may make. When intervening to help a person with an addiction disorder, the clinician must have a sense of the potential contribution of stigma, shame, symptoms, and compromised autonomy in managing not only the disease, but also the psychosocial and ethical repercussions of the disease as experienced by the patient.

The second skill is *the ability to see how one's own life story, attitudes, and knowledge may influence one's care of patients.* What a practitioner assumes to be important regarding quality of life on the basis of his or her own experiences as an athlete, for example, may affect his or her recommendations when providing a consultation for the care of a person who has just survived a serious spinal injury. A corollary to this skill is the clinician's insight about what situations "feel" uncomfortable, which can signal potential patient care conflicts and problems that may be ethical in nature. An example of this type of uncomfortable situation might be an interaction in which a colleague casually requests a prescription for an anxiolytic, wishing not to be formally seen as a patient because of concerns about stigma and being perceived as "weak" by co-workers.

The third skill is *the ability to identify one's areas of clinical expertise* (i.e., scope of clinical competence) *and to work within these boundaries.* This is an ethical skill, because working outside of one's expertise may not serve patients' best interests and may potentially place them in harm's way. The professional obligation in this situation is not to abandon the patient, but instead to ensure that adequate expertise for the patient's care is obtained through consultation or referral. In certain situations, such as in frontier communities, in emergencies, or in training contexts, individuals may ethically perform care outside their scope of competence, but only in response to imperatives to help patients and only with those patients' permission. A related concept is the ethical importance of continuing education so that one's domains of competence remain within community standards, and preferably, the state of the art in broader communities. A second related concept is having a sense of the congruence between one's role (e.g., psychotherapist vs. prison psychiatrist) and the scope and nature of one's ethical obligations.

The fourth skill is *the ability to anticipate ethically risky or problematic situations.* These situations usually pertain to the ethical use of power to ensure the safety of patients or others. Examples include reporting child abuse, committing a patient to an inpatient unit involuntarily, diagnosing substance abuse in an airline pilot or a bus driver, caring for a public official with mental illness, or treating a patient with HIV who does not wish to inform prior sexual partners.

The fifth key ethics skill is ***the ability to gather further information and seek consultation and additional expertise*** in order to clarify and, ideally, to resolve the conflict. This skill may involve reading clinical practice and ethics guidelines, talking with a trusted supervisor, seeking advice from a colleague with specialized expertise, requesting an ethics or a legal consultation, and/or reviewing supplemental clinical data.

The final ethics skill that we wish to emphasize is ***the ability to build additional ethical safeguards into the patient care situation.*** Appropriate use of alternative decision makers, treatment guardians, and advocates may be helpful in caring for a seriously mentally ill individual, for example. Database security firewalls and password-protected computers may be necessary to adequately protect sensitive patient information. Referring patients for confidential treatment off-site may also be necessary in certain circumstances where dual roles and documentation safeguards may infringe upon optimal patient care (e.g., occupational health offices).

These skills represent the basis for ethical practice in mental health care and other clinical fields. They have behavioral components and therefore are observable and potentially measurable. They link directly with the ability to perform certain key activities, such as obtaining informed consent for HIV testing, for example, or speaking with a patient truthfully and responsibly about a medical error and its consequences. For these reasons, these skills will increasingly be incorporated into assessments of the professional and ethical competence of clinicians in coming years.

■ A STRATEGY FOR ETHICAL CLINICAL DECISION MAKING

Clinical ethics is the "identification, analysis, and resolution of moral problems that arise in the care of a particular patient" (Jonsen et al. 1998, p. 3). Clinical ethics centers on everyday choices of caregivers, whether dramatic and extraordinary or mild and mundane. A strategy for approaching and making these sorts of clinical ethics decisions was proposed by Jonsen et al. (1998). It contains four major elements, in their order of importance: 1) clinical indications, 2) preferences of patients, 3) quality of life, and 4) socioeconomic or external factors.

Other medical decision-making models (Table 2–2) have been proposed, although the development of such strategies for psychiatric decision making has been relatively neglected (Roberts et al. 1996). The model of Beauchamp and Childress (2001) is based on the specification and balancing of the four main ethical principles of nonmaleficence, beneficence, autonomy, and justice. Hundert (1987) proffered a technique for identifying "lists of conflicting values" and then using those lists to analyze and resolve the conflicts. Sadler and Hugus (1992) proposed a model in which the core aspects of the clinical encounter—encompassing knowledge, ethics, and pragmatism—are approached in a larger biopsychosocial context as a means of recognizing and processing ethical dilemmas.

TABLE 2–2. **Models of ethical decision-making**

Author	Model	Ethical approach
Jonsen, Siegler, and Winslade	Clinical ethics	Clinical indications Patient preferences Quality of life Contextual factors
Beauchamp and Childress	Balancing and specifying principles	Autonomy Beneficence Nonmaleficence Justice
Hundert	Theoretical framework for conceptualizing moral dilemmas	Lists of conflicting values (e.g., individual freedom vs. safety of the community)
Sadler and Hugus	Clinical encounter within the biopsychosocial context	Knowledge Ethics Pragmatism

Clinical Indications

The first element in the widely applied clinical ethics model proposed by Jonsen et al. (1998) is clinical indications. This element is grounded in the principle of seeking to help and to use all of one's expertise—informed by the body of scientific and practical knowledge of medicine—to serve the well-being and best interests of a patient and to diminish his or her suffering. Clinicians have an obligation to diagnose a patient's condition, to inform and educate the patient about the illness process, to identify and, ordinarily, to recommend optimal options for treatment, and either to carry out those procedures themselves or to ensure that they are carried out by a competent colleague. This first element pertains to the notion of accountability in fulfilling one's responsibility by providing treatment that meets standards of care and is open to scrutiny of colleagues.

Many ethical problems arising in the care of individual patients can be quickly resolved through the application of this first step. For example, in exploring whether an actively suicidal person diagnosed with major depression with psychotic features requires electroconvulsive therapy, the clinician must first examine the severity of the symptoms, the patient's pattern of responsiveness to prior interventions, and the clinical treatment imperatives driven by optimal care standards within the local and national community. Similarly, in debating whether dialysis should be provided for an undocumented immigrant patient or for a patient without appropriate insurance coverage, the first consideration is whether the medical intervention of dialysis is indicated on the basis of clinical knowledge and accepted standards of practice. In this first step of clinical ethics decision making, clinical indications for the individual patient have primacy. Seeking to benefit the individual patient is the imperative within the constraints of what is truly possible within the system of care available and the shared standards of care within the larger community.

Patient Preferences

In keeping with the principle of respect for persons, meaningfully incorporating the preferences of patients is the second step in this decisional process. The importance of this consideration is self-evident, as it helps represent and express the enduring values, voluntarism, and "voice" of the patient. This step is certainly crucial to the therapeutic alliance and to treatment adherence. Nevertheless, especially in the domain of mental illness, incorporating patient preferences can be very complicated. Affective, anxiety, psychotic, and personality disorders alike may be characterized by periods of uncertainty, psychological flux, and cognitive distortions, all of which may influence decisional capacity and the authenticity and stability of expressed choices (Carpenter et al. 2000; Grimes et al. 2000; Roberts 2002). Similarly, end-of-life care preferences in cancer and HIV patients have been shown to be determined more by the adequacy of treatment for pain and depression than by the seriousness or stage of the underlying disease (Bradley et al. 1997; Moser et al. 2002). Cultural beliefs can add an additional layer of complexity; for example, a Native American man may decline a clinically indicated amputation not because he lacks an understanding or appreciation of the seriousness of the situation, but rather because he is concerned that without the amputated tissue he will not be "whole" at the time of his death. In such cases, the patient's objection should be explored and culturally sensitive interventions considered (e.g., inclusion of a native healer who can help find culturally and spiritually acceptable approaches, special preservation of the tissue).

Patient preferences must thus be viewed and interpreted within a clinical framework. In some cases, this consideration will allow the original therapeutic goal to be reached. In other cases, this clinical approach will help the caregiver to see how the wishes expressed by patients may themselves be adversely affected by illness states and to provide appropriate support and treatment. Through such approaches, it is sometimes possible to reach some form of common ground, honoring all imperatives and values in the situation. As discussed in Chapters 4, 5, and 16, respecting the autonomy of patients and their wishes while also fulfilling the responsibilities of recognizing and responding to illness in a manner congruent with accepted standards of care can be quite challenging. Exercising beneficence—seeking to serve the well-being and best interests of patients—without acting paternalistically is very subtle business.

Quality of Life

Quality of life is the third factor that must be taken into account in this model of clinical decision making. Quality of life, although difficult to define, is generally taken to mean the subjective sense of satisfaction expressed and/or experienced by an individual with regard to his or her physical, mental, and social situation (Jonsen et al. 1998). In this step, it is essential to use multiple forms of evidence and, to the greatest extent possible, direct information from the patient's perspective. It is important to note that this step can be very problematic, because it is riddled with assumptions on the part of the clinician. The problematic nature of the quality-of-life factor stems from its reliance on suppositions about both how the ill individual feels and the experiences the individual has undergone in his or her life. When disproportionately emphasized in decision making, the quality-of-life factor may lead to inadequate treatment or to nonbeneficent actions in clinical care. For example, studies of stroke patients and of victims of accidents leading to paralysis suggest that individuals' perceptions of quality of life are determined not by physical deficits but rather by other issues, such as level of pain or degree of disability in some, but not all, activities. The patient's true quality of life, as perceived by the patient him- or herself, may be assessed erroneously by healthy individuals without such physical deficits.

Socioeconomic or External Factors

The fourth and final consideration in this model is socioeconomic or external factors. These factors are diverse and include the interests of society, the role of family members, costs and limitations in access to care, and situational features such as may be present in a research or teaching setting. These features may conflict with one another and with the three prior sets of considerations. For example, the decision to hospitalize a patient may be affected, on the one hand, by the imperative for acute medical intervention, the need to ensure safety for the patient and others, and the desire of a family to have respite and support and, on the other hand, by the patient's expressed desire not to be hospitalized, by his or her lack of insurance, and by the limited number of inpatient beds in the region.

Summary

The use of this strategy is not simple. Like all tools, it offers no guarantees in terms of flawless outcomes. Nevertheless, in conjunction with the set of ethics skills described above, this intentional decision-making strategy may allow the opportunity for systematic reflection and assignment of relative weights to elements that may contribute to the ethical complexity arising in the care of a given patient. Clinicians practicing in the arena of mental health care may find this strategy to be valuable for thinking through cases. With use and adaptation, this decision-making approach may become one of the most helpful and trustworthy of the tools the clinician possesses.

Case Scenarios

A 32-year-old surgeon informs a consulting psychiatrist that he has chosen not to work up an abdominal mass found in a treatment-refractory patient with chronic schizophrenia. When the consultant gently questions the surgeon on his rationale, the surgeon replies that there are "no guarantees" that the mass can be resected or treated. He says that the patient has a "terrible life.... If it is cancer, it will be a blessing."

A 79-year-old man with early dementia refuses a preventive colonoscopy because he does not believe he could handle the surgery and adjunctive treatment. On the basis of this decision, the resident treating the patient insists that the patient "must not" possess decisional capacity. The resident suggests that an alternative decision maker be appointed to approve the procedure; however, the attending physician and the nurse caring for the patient believe that the man's decision-making ability on this issue is intact.

Case Scenarios *(continued)*

A 50-year-old patient with a history of alcohol dependence and bipolar II affective disorder is in psychotherapy. The patient has a history of repeated, near-lethal suicide attempts when severely depressed and intoxicated. He refuses to voluntarily admit himself when his therapist calls him. The case manager states that she will check on him the next day. The psychotherapist arranges for an evaluation at the local psychiatric emergency room and completes the necessary paperwork to have the police collect the patient from his apartment.

The housekeeper at a community health center stops one of the psychiatrists and asks him what to do about his sister, who has been severely depressed ever since she delivered a baby. The psychiatrist requests that the man bring his sister to the psychiatric emergency service and promises that he will arrange for her to be seen. The man shakes his head and says, "She will not come, because she does not have papers, and she is afraid of Immigration."

A 65-year-old woman with recurrent depression has tried many different antidepressants, with only partial response and numerous troubling side effects. After speaking with her psychiatrist, she decides to try electroconvulsive therapy. Her children become very upset and call the psychiatrist, telling him that their mother's decision must be a sign that she wants to die.

■ REFERENCES

Beauchamp TL, Childress JF: Principles of Biomedical Ethics, 5th Edition. New York, Oxford University Press, 2001

Bradley E, Walker L, Blechner B, et al: Assessing capacity to participate in discussions of advance directives in nursing homes: findings from a study of the Patient Self Determination Act. J Am Geriatr Soc 45:79–83, 1997

Carpenter WT Jr, Gold JM, Lahti AC, et al: Decisional capacity for informed consent in schizophrenia research [see comments]. Arch Gen Psychiatry 57:533–538, 2000

Grimes AL, McCullough LB, Kunik ME, et al: Informed consent and neuroanatomic correlates of intentionality and voluntariness among psychiatric patients. Psychiatr Serv 51:1561–1567, 2000

Hundert EM: A model for ethical problem solving in medicine, with practical applications. Am J Psychiatry 144:839–846, 1987

Jonsen AR, Siegler M, Winslade WJ: Clinical Ethics, 4th Edition. New York, McGraw-Hill, 1998

Morenz B, Sales B: Complexity of ethical decision making in psychiatry. Ethics Behav 7(1):1–14, 1997

Moser DJ, Schultz SK, Arndt S, et al: Capacity to provide informed consent for participation in schizophrenia and HIV research. Am J Psychiatry 159:1201–1207, 2002

Roberts LW: Informed consent and the capacity for voluntarism. Am J Psychiatry 159:705–712, 2002

Roberts LW, McCarty T, Roberts BB, et al: Clinical ethics teaching in psychiatric supervision. Acad Psychiatry 20:172–184, 1996

Sadler JZ, Hulgus YF: Clinical problem solving and the biopsychosocial model. Am J Psychiatry 149:1315–1323, 1992

3

THE PSYCHOTHERAPEUTIC
RELATIONSHIP

Immanuel Kant once observed, "We are not gentleman volunteers; we are conscripts in the army of moral law" (Murdoch 1992, p. 35). We recognize that many individuals act primarily, perhaps exclusively, in self-interest. But Kant's observation that there is a moral imperative—what he called a "categorical imperative"—is indeed compelling. We cannot ignore the fact that moral demands are placed upon us by virtue of our living in a social order with other human beings.

Physicians and health professionals in particular live in a moral order, with obligations incumbent on them by virtue of the needs of those who seek their help. Acknowledging that there are scoundrels among professionals, those motivated solely by self-interest and not in the service of others, we recognize that there are certain demands that health professionals cannot escape. Specific moral obligations are imposed on them by virtue of their relationship with patients or clients. This relationship is shaped by the clinician's promise and expertise to heal and by the imbalance that naturally exists between a person in need and a person who seeks to provide treatment, answers, and comfort in relation to that need. Whether one understands those obligations as allegiance to conscience, allegiance to God, allegiance to society, or a more direct allegiance to the patient or client, the obligations are present.

■ PROFESSIONALISM IN THE PSYCHOTHERAPEUTIC RELATIONSHIP

The relationship of clinician and patient is sometimes spoken of as a sacred trust. That bond deserves further reflection and careful understanding. A fiduciary relationship means a relationship of trust. Law understands fiduciary differently from medicine and other clinical fields. In law a fiduciary, or trustee, may act on behalf of the client. In the health professions, the trust derives from the relationship and must be earned again and again in every moment. The clinician acts with the patient in true partnership.

In the early years when bioethics began to emerge as a discipline distinct from medical ethics, a question was often posed, "Is there anything distinct about medical ethics, or is it just everyday ethics applied to medical situations?" (Clouser 1974). The more mature discipline of *biomedical ethics* recognizes multiple perspectives (physician/professional, patient/client, and society) on what goes on in this very special and personal encounter. These diverse perspectives offer valuable insights into the relationship.

Since the early 1980s, many professionals have spoken of this relationship as a relationship with a client, suggesting a more explicit, business-oriented contract with a more or less coequal autonomous person. Such a relationship implies more responsibility for the client, consistent with more contemporary notions of autonomy, but no less responsibility for the professional. And whereas physicians once understood their obligations almost exclusively in terms of a principle of beneficence, and still do, it would never be permissible to act with a disregard for the patient's wishes and needs, although those may at times be in conflict.

Over the past 24 centuries, the Hippocratic writings (Oath, Corpus, Aphorisms) have placed special obligations on physicians that were not incumbent on members of society in general. For example, the proscription against sex with patients ("mischief") applied to physicians in a unique way in ancient Greek society. As an itinerant healer, the physician might spend extended periods in a particular household. It would not be unusual in that society for the master of the house to provide sexual companions to a guest. Physicians, followers of the Oath, set themselves apart from this practice, no doubt with a sense that their function in the household was not as a recipient of hospitality and with recognition that indulging in their own comforts would compromise their effectiveness.

Much of the understanding and misunderstanding about the therapeutic relationship involves the recognition of a sexual or sexualized tension between therapist and patient/client. Even when sex does not occur, there may be sexualized feelings and fantasies. Distinctions are important, and subtleties are important. The clinician comes into contact with people at a time of vulnerability imposed by the illness. In order for the clinician to be able to understand the patient's illness, the patient must subject him- or herself to a degree of scrutiny not encountered elsewhere in life. The patient must be examined physically and psychologically—exposed, unclothed, naked, vulnerable. The patient, a person seeking care, must disclose the most personal information imaginable—indeed, information that one might not readily imagine as possible to discuss with another. Ancient traditions (Hippocrates as the most ready example) recognized the imperative that such information be kept confidential, private, and secret within the relationship ("not noised abroad"). Professionals have vigorously stood by this principle for millennia, holding that therapeutic work could not take place without the guarantee of that privacy. Certain situations are recognized in which it may be permissible or even mandatory to violate this secrecy, such as when child abuse is suspected or the risk of violence is present. Even when such disclosures may be mandated by the state (i.e., government, court, or law), however, they are never made without regard for confidentiality—the confidence and trust of the patient.

Confidentiality, understood as trust, is a value that is gradually being eroded in modern health care. Medical information is shared between practitioners only with the explicit consent of the patient/client. However, insurance companies freely share pooled information about every claim, provider encounter, diagnosis, and treatment. This is done under a blanket consent, which everyone signs when applying for insurance. Although the consent is tacitly recognized, it is really a coerced consent. One could not use insurance without giving consent for review of records. Perhaps most disturbing in this trend is the recent federal privacy guidelines, which eliminate formal requirements for patients to consent specifically and prospectively to the use of their medical information. Indeed, under the new guidelines, personal medical information no longer belongs to the patient.

Psychotherapists are the first to sound the alarm and cry "foul." True therapy cannot occur without the assurance of privacy. One could not feel free to talk to a therapist (and certainly not about personal matters) if it were known or suspected that such information might be shared with others. Such information could be misused by employers or might be used at some future time to prevent employment or discriminate against the consumer—for example, in obtaining health insurance. Ethics in such considerations is not just a matter of personal conscience for the provider; it is also a matter of social policy, law, and respect for and protection of individual rights.

The solely commercial understanding of the patient undermines the understanding professional relationship as an ethical commitment to the suffering person. Commercial expediency cannot be good for our society. Healing calls upon a more universal good. It invokes the sacred. It invokes the ability to appeal to another in a community with the trust that such an appeal will bring needed help. The healer understands that appeal not just as a participant in a commercial transaction, but also as a member of a caring community.

■ THE NATURE OF THE PSYCHOTHERAPEUTIC ENCOUNTER

In this commercial era, the therapeutic encounter is often thought of as an exchange of commodity—a pill, a procedure. More basically, the therapeutic encounter encompasses all that transpires between doctor and patient (professional–client), including especially talking, listening, telling one's story, biography, medical "history," examination (often including a physical exam), evaluation, counseling, treatment planning, follow-up, reconsideration, recommendations, and more follow-up. Many ancient and contemporary traditions view the medical practitioner as a shamanistic healer—someone who has magical powers, someone who can harmonize the spirits; the person to whom a sick person turns for help is someone who can be believed in because of the powers he or she commands. This is no different today in our society, when the powers believed in are understood to be medical technologies, a complex body of information, much of which is arcane, most of which is believed and hoped to be useful.

The relationship between the sick and the healer has received the most scrutiny in the psychoanalytic tradition—psychoanalysis and the derivative psychotherapies. The therapeutic relationship is best understood in this encounter, which is essentially little different from the encounter with the stereotyped brusque surgeon or with the mysterious shaman—except for the scrutiny given to the relationship itself.

It was Sigmund Freud's particular genius to recognize that when two people spend time together, they develop feelings that derive from other significant relationships in their prior experience. Significantly, the patient develops feelings for the physician that repeat feelings held for parents. Freud called this phenomenon *transference* and recognized that it could be a vehicle for understanding past experience. It is beyond the scope of this book to assess the place of Freudian theory in psychotherapy, but an appreciation of the concept of transference is essential for understanding the ethics of the therapeutic relationship.

Psychotherapists structure a frame within which the reflective process can occur. They agree to meet at a certain time at a certain place for a certain duration at a certain frequency for a certain purpose. These are the boundaries of the frame and the boundaries of the therapeutic relationship. Development of a therapeutic alliance is part of the therapy in which the patient allies with the clinician to get better. More specifically, the part of the patient that wants to get better allies with the therapist to understand the part of the patient that wants to repeat maladaptive behavior patterns. This repetition is called *resistance*. In the early years of psychoanalysis, resistance was seen as an obstacle that needed to be overcome before analysis could be successful. Today, resistance is appreciated more sympathetically as part of a defense structure that must be accepted and understood. Too-rigid adherence to the boundaries places the therapist at risk of appearing uncaring and of increasing the patient's defenses. Disregard of the boundaries compromises the therapist's chances of creating a situation in which reflection can occur. The therapist walks a delicate tightrope, demonstrating concern and empathy yet insisting on scrutinizing what takes place between clinician and patient as a possible transference clue that needs to be understood.

The case examples that follow illustrate everyday dilemmas that can be problematic as matters of technique, judgment, and ethics.

Case 1

A woman approached therapy eagerly and with energy. She was polite, easygoing, and friendly. She was interested in the therapist, curious about the therapists' personal life, and, in a social way, asked ordinary but persistent questions, such as "Did you have a nice vacation? Where did you go?" The therapist recognized these questions as a departure from the therapeutic stance, but he felt that it would be too much work to keep inquiring about the curiosity behind the questions, when in fact they were innocent enough.

This ordinary situation is one that every therapist encounters. How is the frame established? Should the therapeutic frame be set when the patient is met in the waiting room, when the door to the consulting room is closed, or when the patient settles down and begins to work? How should chance encounters be handled? What if patient and therapist are thrown together in some community activity, as is especially likely to happen in small communities? The Exploitation Index, an educational tool developed by Epstein and Simon (1990; Epstein et al. 1992) for use in examining therapeutic boundary issues, provides an opportunity to consider some of the situations in which boundary crossings or frank transgressions may be an unrecognized issue (see Appendix to this chapter).

Most therapists encounter such situations, which can be quite awkward and which require a certain discipline to remind the patient that therapy is different from a social relationship and to hold the therapeutic frame.

Case 2

A young woman consulted a psychiatrist for help with anxiety and disappointment with relationships with men. She was open, energetic, talkative, and highly successful in her profession. The psychiatrist considered himself a "medical psychopharmacologist" and prescribed an appropriate medication for this patient. He was in fact skeptical of psychotherapeutic approaches to dealing with problems he knew could respond quickly to medication. He saw nothing wrong with an extraprofessional relationship that did not involve dating or physical intimacy, so he accepted the patient's invitations to her pool parties. Although he considered this just being sociable, the patient felt that more was involved and understood.

Although this clinician had not crossed the boundary into a sexual relationship, he failed to appreciate the boundary that he should have recognized between a professional relationship and a social relationship.

Case 3

A young man sought therapy because of disappointments in his life. He felt that his therapist was someone who understood and cared for him, and he looked forward to their sessions. When he became particularly distressed, the therapist would schedule him as the last appointment of the day and sometimes would extend the sessions. The therapist felt that supportive therapy was indicated and that the patient needed support to face the difficulties in his life. When the therapist later began to limit the time in the sessions, the patient became hurt and angry and decided to end the treatment, because he felt it was no longer working.

These cases share ordinariness; they are common situations in therapy that offer dilemmas and raise questions of values. They are matters of technique and judgment. No deliberate harm was done, although opportunities for good might have been missed. Often, therapists will say that they do not deal with the transference; that is an issue for psychoanalysis. But as these mundane examples illustrate, transference feelings can arise in all kinds of therapy.

Clear boundary violations, such as sex with a patient or failure to maintain confidentiality, are obviously unethical and can be devastating for the patient as a personal violation of trust. The proscription against sex with a patient is clear and unambiguous in the codes of ethics of all professions. The American Psychiatric Association's (2001) *Principles of Medical Ethics With Annotations Especially Applicable to Psychiatry* explicitly state that sexual activity with a patient is unethical.

Case 4

A medical student was threatened with expulsion from medical school when it was discovered that he had had sex with a patient on the service where he was rotating. When the matter was brought to administrative attention, the student stated in his own defense that the sex was "consensual" and that he had not realized that there was anything wrong with it: "It wasn't like it happened on the psychiatry rotation, or anything like that."

Sexual relations with patients (and former patients) receives the closest scrutiny in psychiatry and in psychotherapeutic relations, but the same transferential concerns of trust, dependency, and idealization occur in other professional relationships as well.

What about sex with a former patient? Is that ever permissible? Are the expectations different for a relationship with a patient who is seen once on a consultative basis and a patient who is involved in a psychotherapeutic relationship? Might it be possible after a specified period of time—say, 1 or 2 years—to engage in a personal, intimate, sexual relationship with a person who was formerly a patient? And if so, how could it be determined what the appropriate "cooling off" period should be? The American Psychiatric Association has taken an increasingly austere stance on this issue. Whereas the statement in the 1973 version of *The Principles of Medical Ethics* read, "Sex with a current patient is unethical. Sex with a former patient is almost always unethical" (American Psychiatric Association 1973, p. 4), that annotation was revised in 1993, and in all iterations published since then, the statement is absolutely unequivocal: "Sexual activity with a current or former patient is unethical" (American Psychiatric Association 2001, Section 2, Annotation 1). It is possible that a physician and a patient could truly fall in love and commit themselves to each other forever. But should the relationship subsequently turn sour, the patient (or former patient) could always claim exploitation on the part of the physician.

We have spoken of boundary violations as transgressions primarily in the frame of the psychotherapeutic relationship. This is the easiest way to grasp the concept of boundaries, but in fact boundaries are more complicated in everyday life. The boundary that the therapist must respect is the boundary between self and other, between therapist and patient. That is a complicated boundary because, like other relationships, it has a transference component. The extent to which a patient may wish to please (or to rebel against) the therapist may be a repetition of feelings developed in childhood in relationship to significant others. Parents who used their children to gratify their own wishes probably left those children vulnerable to exploitation by others. Such children are said to have been used as narcissistic extensions of their parents. In the extreme form of this problem, the boundary between parent and child is not established, and the exploitation may be perverse. But the successful student or athlete may be working for the pride of the parent rather than a sense of personal accomplishment, a pride that may be inadvertently exploited by a teacher or coach with the best of intentions. The effective and ethical therapist works to establish and maintain a boundary that—despite often appearing artificial at first—eventually provides the emotional distance for the patient to develop an autonomous sense of self. This sense of self expands the philosophical concept of autonomy that is so important to bioethics.

With an appreciation of the transference dynamics of the boundary between therapist and patient, self and other, and of the practical ethical consequences of this boundary's violation, it is possible to look at the question of a relationship with a former patient in a new light. From the standpoint of an enduring commitment, we may recognize marriage as the possible exception to the "never" rule. With the recognition of transference feelings, however, we caution therapists that the partner may later claim that the feelings once understood as love were in actuality a transference that was exploited in therapy. It would be very difficult indeed to defend oneself against such a claim.

Several considerations can help clarify the understanding of boundaries:

- *Nonsexual boundary violations*—Sexual boundaries and boundary violations receive the most attention because their violations are the most devastating. But if the violations are understood to represent a transgression of self and other, there are also other aspects of the relationship that can be transgressed—for example, business, financial, religious, and social.
- *Boundary crossings*—Sometimes a therapist will experience an internal sense of discomfort at having allowed him- or herself or the patient to cross a certain boundary. The transgressions may be minor self-disclosures (e.g., talking about vacations or one's personal life), extratherapeutic social encounters, or just a sense that one is not holding the therapeutic frame. Although unlikely to result in formal ethics complaints, such boundary crossings may undermine the clinician's ability to do effective therapy. Recognition of a boundary transgression should prompt the therapist to seek consultation or supervision or to reflect on his or her motives in personal therapy. If the therapist is a trainee, it is the task of the supervisor to create an environment in which such self-awareness can occur and to help the trainee come to an appropriate resolution. Sometimes boundary crossings can illuminate the transference–countertransference dynamic and thereby further therapeutic understanding.

- *Divided loyalties*—Situations occur in therapy when the therapist experiences divided loyalties—allegiance to the patient as well as allegiance to some other interest (Knight 1995). These situations have traditionally been spoken of as the "dual agent" problem. A physician or therapist is a dual agent, for example, if he or she owes an allegiance to his or her employer as well as to the patient. A classic example of this dilemma is the psychiatrist or psychologist working for the military or for a state or federal institution. Increasing numbers of physicians and other providers are now working for large organizations, such as health maintenance organizations or managed care companies, rather than in independent practices. Subtler issues involving overlapping and divided loyalty arise for small-community clinicians, who must serve not only their individual patients but also their patients' families, who are neighbors and friends (see Chapter 10). More globally, clinicians increasingly recognize an allegiance to society, which makes it increasingly difficult to buffer a unique concern for each individual patient.

More extreme cases put the more mundane cases into perspective. Psychiatrists in the former Soviet Union, as well as in other Eastern European countries and in the People's Republic of China, have come under scrutiny for hospitalizing political dissidents and labeling them mentally ill or "psychiatrically impaired" (Lifton 1976). Physicians in the military governments in Latin American and in several African nations have (perhaps under coercion themselves) cooperated with torture of political prisoners. Nazi physicians conducted experiments in concentration camps, which would previously have been unimaginable and which have given rise to many safeguards in human research (Lifton 1986).

From a moral perspective, most double-agent situations are best seen as cases of conflicting loyalty or clashing duties. The clinician must choose one duty over another (Macklin 1982). Perhaps most problematic are situations in which the patient assumes (because of the weight of the professions' patient-centered ethic) that the clinician is working exclusively for the patient's best interests and well-being. Thus, a psychiatrist conducting a prearraignment examination might be able to elicit more information than a police interrogator simply by projecting a trustworthy demeanor. But if the message is not "I am here to help you," then the purpose of the examination should be directly stated. A therapist conducting an administrative evaluation in a student health service should clearly state, "You are being evaluated at the request of the Dean, who will receive a report of my findings." A mental health professional should not convey the impression that everything discussed will be confidential if that is not the case. In clinical research, the issue of dual agency ("the therapeutic misconception") has become recognized as a key ethical consideration (see Chapter 16).

Furthermore, review and examination of double-agent issues should be a continuing obligation of mental health professionals, for such scrutiny is the only way to prevent such issues from disrupting the clinician–client relationship. These are issues that often come before professional ethics committees and serve as reminders of the ethical principles kept alive through education, codes, and professional discipline.

When a conflict of interest arises, the health care professional should make his or her allegiance to the patient/client primary and should fully inform the patient/client of the conflict of interest. The goal of maintaining trust is essential to the therapeutic relationship, and anything that erodes that goal diminishes not only the therapy, but also the therapist and the profession he or she represents.

Case Scenarios

A psychology intern completing a rotation in the rape crisis clinic notices a classmate from her training program in the waiting room; the classmate is coming in for crisis evaluation and treatment after an assault the night before.

The chair of psychiatry at an academic medical center receives a call from the CEO of the university hospital, requesting mental health treatment for her mother-in-law.

Case Scenarios *(continued)*

A psychotherapist attending a small dinner party discovers that one of the other dinner guests is a client of his.

A psychiatrist routinely encounters one of his patients at a coffee shop near his office. The patient appears to be waiting for him there and often tries to engage him in conversations that are intensely personal.

A young, married psychiatry resident begins caring for a patient who has many sexual partners. He finds himself becoming very curious about the new sexual liaisons of the patient and very much looks forward to each therapy session with this patient.

A consultation-liaison psychiatrist with duties at a community hospital receives a psychiatric referral for a patient who was recently diagnosed with testicular cancer. She has known the patient for several years, and they went on a "casual date" 4 years ago.

■ REFERENCES

American Psychiatric Association: The Principles of Medical Ethics With Annotations Applicable to Psychiatry. Washington, DC, American Psychiatric Association, 2001

Clouser KD: What is medical ethics? Ann Intern Med 80:657–660, 1974

Epstein RS, Simon RI: The Exploitation Index: an early warning indicator of boundary violations in psychotherapy. Bull Menninger Clin 54:450–465, 1990

Epstein RS, Simon RI, Kay GG: Assessing boundary violations in psychotherapy: survey results with the Exploitation Index. Bull Menninger Clin 56:150–166, 1992

Knight JA: Divided loyalties in mental health care, in Encyclopedia of Bioethics, 2nd Edition. Reich WT, Editor-in-Chief. New York, Macmillan, 1995, pp 629–633

Lifton RJ: Advocacy and corruption in the healing professions. International Review of Psychoanalysis 3(4):385–398, 1976

Lifton RJ: The Nazi Doctors: Medical Killing and the Psychology of Genocide. New York, Basic Books, 1986

Macklin R: Man, Mind, and Morality: The Ethics of Behavior Control. Englewood Cliffs, NJ, Prentice Hall, 1982

Murdoch I: Metaphysics as a Guide to Morals: Philosophical Reflections. New York, Viking Penguin, 1992

Appendix

THE EXPLOITATION INDEX

Rate yourself according to the frequency that the following statements reflect your behavior, thoughts, or feelings with regard to any particular patients you have seen in psychotherapy within the past 2 years, by placing a check in the appropriate box. Approximate frequency as follows:

- Never
- Rarely = Once a year or less
- Sometimes = About once every 3 months
- Often = Once a month or more

Please give your immediate, "off the cuff" responses:

	Never	Rarely	Some- times	Often
1. Do you do any of the following for your family members or social acquaintances: prescribing medication, making diagnoses, offering psychodynamic explanations for their behavior?				
2. Are you gratified by a sense of power when you are able to control a patient's activity through advice, medication, or behavioral restraint (e.g., hospitalization, seclusion)?				
3. Do you find the chronic silence or tardiness of a patient a satisfying way of getting paid for doing nothing?				
4. Do you accept gifts or bequests from patients?				
5. Have you engaged in a personal relationship with a patient after treatment was terminated?				

The Exploitation Index *(continued)*

	Never	Rarely	Some-times	Often
6. Do you touch your patients (exclude handshake)?				
7. Do you ever use information learned from patients, such as business tips or political information, for your own financial or career gain?				
8. Do you feel that you can obtain personal gratification by helping to develop your patient's great potential for fame or unusual achievement?				
9. Do you feel a sense of excitement or longing when you think of a patient or anticipate her/his visit?				
10. Do you make exceptions for your patients, such as providing special scheduling or reducing fees, because you find the patient attractive, appealing, or impressive?				
11. Do you ask your patient to do personal favors for you (e.g., get you lunch, mail a letter)?				
12. Do you and your patients address each other on a first-name basis?				
13. Do you undertake business deals with patients?				
14. Do you take great pride in the fact that such an attractive, wealthy, powerful, or important patient is seeking your help?				
15. Have you accepted for treatment persons with whom you have had social involvement or whom you knew to be in your social or family sphere?				

APPENDIX   **The Exploitation Index** *(continued)*

	Never	Rarely	Some-times	Often
16. When your patient has been seductive with you, do you experience this as a gratifying sign of your own scx appeal?				
17. Do you disclose sensational aspects of your patient's life to others (even when you are protecting the patient's identity)?				
18. Do you accept a medium of exchange other than money for your services (e.g., work on your office or home, trading of professional services)?				
19. Do you find yourself comparing the gratifying qualities you observe in a patient with the less-gratifying qualities in your spouse or significant other (e.g., thinking "where have you been all my life?")?				
20. Do you feel that your patient's problems would be immeasurably helped if only he/she had a positive romantic involvement with you?				
21. Do you make exceptions in the conduct of treatment because you feel sorry for your patient, or because you believe that he/she is in such distress or so disturbed that you have no other choice?				
22. Do you recommend treatment procedures or referrals that you do not believe to be necessarily in your patient's best interests, but that may instead be to your direct or indirect financial benefit?				

The Exploitation Index *(continued)*

	Never	Rarely	Some-times	Often
23. Have you accepted for treatment individuals known to be referred by a current or former patient?				
24. Do you make exceptions for your patient because you are afraid she/he will otherwise become extremely angry or self-destructive?				
25. Do you take pleasure in romantic daydreams about a patient?				
26. Do you fail to deal with the following patient behavior(s): paying the fee late, missing appointments on short notice and refusing to pay for the time (as agreed), seeking to extend the length of sessions?				
27. Do you tell patients personal things about yourself in order to impress them?				
28. Do you find yourself trying to influence your patients to support political causes or positions in which you have a personal interest?				
29. Do you seek social contact with patients outside of clinically scheduled visits?				
30. Do you find it painfully difficult to agree to a patient's desire to cut down on the frequency of therapy, or to work on termination?				
31. Do you find yourself talking about your own personal problems with a patient and expecting her/him to be sympathetic to you?				

APPENDIX   **The Exploitation Index** *(continued)*

	Never	*Rarely*	*Some-times*	*Often*
32. Do you join in any activity with a patient that may serve to deceive a third party (e.g., an insurance company)?				

Scoring Key: Never = 0, Rarely = 1, Sometimes = 2, Often = 3. A total score of 27 or greater would compare to the highest 10% as found in a pilot study with a sample of 532 psychiatrists.

Source.   Reprinted from Epstein RS, Simon RI: "The Exploitation Index: An Early Warning Indicator of Boundary Violations in Psychotherapy." *Bulletin of the Menninger Clinic* 54:450–465, 1990. Used with permission.

INFORMED CONSENT AND DECISIONAL CAPACITY

Informed consent is a philosophical and legal doctrine that has come to serve as the cornerstone of ethically sound clinical care in our society. Informed consent requires that an individual truly understand and freely make a decision to undertake—or not—a proposed treatment approach in light of his or her own personal health care goals. Informed consent emphasizes respect for the individual, and it is inherently relational—that is, it occurs in the context of a professional relationship. In this chapter, we describe the core elements of informed consent in clinical care (Figure 4–1). Differing standards for consent, advance directives and surrogate decision making, empirical studies related to consent, and constructive approaches to the process of informed consent are surveyed as well.

■ ELEMENTS OF INFORMED CONSENT

The Therapeutic Relationship

Consent occurs in a context, both institutional and interpersonal. Consent is obtained in jail psychiatric units, in community clinics, and on hospital wards by physicians, nurses, social workers, and other health professionals. In all of these circumstances and in all of these relationships, fulfilling the concept of informed consent in clinical care means that concern for promoting the health and alleviating the suffering of the individual patient will be the absolute basis of any recommended treatment. This is true regardless of whether the relationship involves a brief encounter to refill a pa-

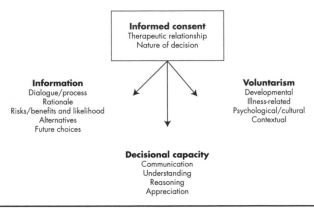

FIGURE 4–1. **Elements of informed consent.**

tient's medications in a busy walk-in clinic, a problem-focused consultation by a specialist on a hospital ward, or intensive therapy sessions over many years. The clinician's dedication to the health, well-being, and best interests of the patient is embodied in this relationship. It gives emphasis to the patient's personal values and the overall goals for the patient's care. It is characterized by compassion, trust, and honesty. In research consent, the relationship continues to be characterized by these qualities, but there is a balance between the needs of the patient and the needs of the scientific endeavor, as described in Chapter 16.

Information

The sharing of appropriate information is the second of the four core elements of informed consent. The patient should be provided with accurate and balanced information regarding the anticipated risks and benefits of a given treatment and its alternatives and their expected outcomes. Alternatives may include implementation of another treatment or of additional treatment, or it may involve no intervention in the course of illness at all. For example, in obtaining informed consent for treatment of mild depression, the clinician should discuss the variable course of depressive illnesses, including the potential for symptom resolution in the absence of treatment. In this discussion, the clinician should review the rationale for a proposed antidepressant agent, given the symptoms of the patient (e.g., obsessionality, psychotic features, insomnia, agitation) and the attitudes and values of the patient (e.g., fears about being "dependent" on a medication, concerns related to sexual functioning or weight gain, individual preferences for psychosocial treatments, culturally influenced interpretations of personal symptoms). The discussion should cover the medication's possible side effects, potential adverse effects, and their relative likelihood. Alternative approaches to treatment should also be discussed in light of their merit for an individual patient who is depressed. Insight-oriented, interpersonal, and supportive therapies, electroconvulsive therapy (ECT), light therapy, "natural" approaches (e.g., herbal remedies, St. John's wort, vitamins), placebo effects, and nontreatment are topics that may arise in this discussion.

Determining how much detail to offer about a specific treatment approach and its alternatives can sometimes be difficult. A few "rules of thumb" are useful in making this judgment. It is good to start with a "reasonable person" standard—that is, what would a reasonable person need to know in order to make this decision? For example, in obtaining consent for initiation of a psychotropic medication, such as carbamazepine, it is important to explain the utility of serum levels and the potential effects of the medication on the patient's liver and bone marrow. Decreased white blood cell counts and increased vulnerability to infection are not so rare that they should be omitted, and the predictable hepatic metabolism changes should be explained so that necessary adjustments in other medications can be anticipated and understood by the patient. Such information may need to be offered in increments, and additional information about the specific treatment rationale may be appropriate for some patients. In some cases, less information may be necessary, but in no case should the aim in omitting data be to deceive or mislead the patient so that he or she will accept the offered treatment.

Decisional Capacity

Decisional capacity, the third element of informed consent, represents a sophisticated clinical assessment of an individual's global and specific cognitive abilities within a particular context (Appelbaum and Grisso 1988). Such an assessment can be a very subtle and complex exercise. Decisional capacity must be understood according to the type of decision to be made; the enduring, emerging, and fluctuating attributes of the individual; the nature and severity of the person's symptoms; the precise nature of the patient's situation; his or her prior experiences, personal values, psychological defenses, and coping style; and other factors.

The presence of a serious symptom (e.g., delusions, memory loss, suicidal ideation, diminished cognitive functioning) or of a serious diagnosis (e.g., schizophrenia, dementia, major depression, developmental disability) does *not* mean that an individual lacks decisional capacity. Similarly, being a young child or a very elderly person does *not,* a priori, preclude one from being decisionally capable (see Chapter 7). In addition, it should be noted that decisional capacity is a clinical assessment. It is distinct from "competence," which is a legal determination—that is, a formal assessment by a judge or other officer of the court regarding a person's ability to function within a particular domain of life (e.g., financial decisions, treatment decisions).

Decisional capacity has four principal components, each of which should be viewed on a continuum and not as an "all or nothing" phenomenon. The first component is the individual's ability to express a preference (i.e., capacity for expression of choice or for communication). On the extreme end of the continuum will be severely ill psychiatric patients who are mute or catatonic, or who manifest complete language and thought disorganization (e.g., "word salad"), for instance, and therefore are "incapable" of communication. In the medical context, a patient who is comatose due to metabolic disturbances, aphasic secondary to a stroke, or unconscious after a head injury will also lack this first, most fundamental ability. Individuals who have periods of altered consciousness in delirium may be intermittently incapable of communication. Depressed patients who are so severely ill that they do not speak or care for themselves often may be deemed decisionally incapable simply because they do not make clear their preferences, either through language or action. At times this component of decisional capacity is very difficult to assess, such as in a patient with spinal cord injury who can communicate only through eye blinks or a stroke patient with Broca's aphasia who is overwhelmed and frustrated by the process of generating words. For these reasons, although the ability to express a preference is often obvious, in many situations this assessment will require careful interactions with patients and astute observational and listening skills on the part of the clinician.

The second component of decisional capacity is the individual's ability to understand relevant information (i.e., capacity for comprehension). In talking with the clinician, the patient with this ability will be able to take in factual information regarding the nature of the illness, the need for intervention, the kinds of treatments under consideration, their relative risks and benefits, and the possible consequences of not intervening with treatment. Depending on the patient's illness, comorbid conditions, potential therapeutic options, and educational level, this information may be relatively straightforward or highly complicated. In assessing this element of decisional capacity, it is critical that the patient state his or her understanding of the situation and the choices at hand in his or her own words. Otherwise, it is difficult to know whether the patient is using terms and phrases of the clinicians without truly understanding their meaning and implications.

Third is the individual's ability to think through the choice at hand in a way that is "rational" and deliberate (i.e., capacity for reasoning or rational thinking). This component of decisional capacity—which I refer to as the "Spock criterion" when teaching my students (who invariably are Star Trek fans)—relates to the person's analytical abilities given a specific set of facts or data. For instance, the rational person, all other factors being equal, will consistently choose a medication that has a 75% likelihood of treating the illness effectively over one that has a 50% likelihood. Similarly, the rational person, all other factors being equal, will consistently choose the medication that poses the fewest risks and promises the fewest adverse side effects. In essence, this dimension of decisional capacity has to do with the ability to use information in what is considered to be an objective manner. However, this does not mean that the individual must choose the "rational thing" when making a treatment decision; rather, it is the person's ability to see the reasons for and against a given option in the larger setting of his or her life.

Fourth, and often most importantly, is the person's ability to make meaning of the decision and its consequences within the context of his or her personal history, values, emotions, and life situation (i.e., capacity for appreciation). Deeply dependent on psychological insight, this component is in our opinion the most sophisticated element of decisional capacity. It can be very difficult to assess clinically. For instance, some individuals with early dementia have relatively intact social and cognitive skills and yet are unable to think through the meaning of an important treatment decision and its repercussions. Similarly, in certain patients with mental disorders, the negative cognitive distortions caused by the illness may interfere with their ability to interpret information within a personal context. This has been demonstrated in the work of Ganzini et al. (1994), who found that the end-of-life care preferences of severely depressed inpatients may be shaped by their negative expectations of the future, guilt, self-blame, and dysphoria, all of which are attributable to their mental illness, not to their authentic and stable beliefs and values. After treatment, these same individuals made significantly more positive care choices (e.g., desire for life-preserving interventions, predictions of likely outcomes of these interventions) when they envisioned the future.

Consider two examples related to the decision to amputate an infected foot. A patient with insulin-dependent diabetes mellitus, a seriously infected lesion on the sole of his foot, and multi-infarct dementia was seen on the consultation-liaison psychiatry service because of concerns about his ability to make a decision about possible amputation. He was capable of stating the reasons for the recommended procedure, and he appeared to agree with this recommendation, but he did not really understand that amputation meant that he would actually lose his foot permanently, that he would require a prosthesis in his shoe, that he would receive physical therapy, or that the surgery might not be successful in containing the infection and that another surgery might be required to preserve the functioning of his leg. He also did not understand that he could die if the infection progressed and were not treated aggressively. This was not a simple issue of poor communication, inadequate information, or poor understanding of factual information; all of these things had been explained to him by different individuals on various occasions, and multiple scenarios depicting treatment outcomes had been discussed with him. He had listened attentively, and he could repeat the information back and apparently state the "rational" implications of this information to the clinician. Nevertheless, he could not apply the meaning of the surgery to his own life situation, present or future.

In contrast, a Navajo man with diabetes and an infected foot seen on the consultation-liaison service was evaluated because he had refused amputation. The treatment team felt that he was being "irrational." In this case, the patient was able to communicate and to understand the need for the procedure and the full ramifications of declining the procedure, and he still elected to continue with antibiotic therapies, which previously had met with little success. In this case, the patient was a very traditional Navajo, and he was clear that the amputation was too dangerous spiritually and psychologically in the absence of a native healer. His desire was to delay the procedure, not refuse it altogether, on the grounds that he appreciated what the true impact of the decision would be for him if the amputation were performed in a manner that was not congruent with his culture.

In sum, appreciation is the dimension of decisional capacity in which personal values are integrated with expressive, factual, and rational data and processes within the real context of the individual patient's life.

Voluntarism

Beyond information and decisional capacity, the final element of informed consent is voluntarism (Roberts 2002). Voluntarism encompasses the individual's ability to act in accord with his or her authentic sense of what is good, right, and best in light of his or her situation, values, and prior history. Voluntarism further entails the capacity to make this choice freely and in the absence of coercion. Deliberateness, purposefulness of intent, clarity, genuineness, and coherence with prior life decisions are important to voluntarism. Voluntarism thus represents the manifestation of the autonomous, authentic preferences of the individual. Autonomous wishes may be deeply influenced by social and cultural expectations and psychological history. For instance, a patient who has been in the military may be oriented to hierarchical power relationships and may view a clinician's recommendation as an "order" to be obeyed. Similarly, a patient who has been a victim of violence may see herself as relatively powerless, and a patient who has been institutionalized involuntarily in the past may see himself as no longer possessing the right to his own views. In sum, voluntary preferences may be tempered by the realities of the situation (e.g., the presence of a serious diagnosis, the lack of "curative" treatments for many mental illnesses) but should reflect the person's genuine wishes in the absence of external coercion (e.g., pressure by an employer not to seek mental health care).

Voluntarism may be understood as being influenced in four areas: 1) developmental factors; 2) illness-related considerations; 3) psychological issues and cultural and religious values; and 4) external features and pressures. In terms of developmental factors, it is clear that a person's capacity for voluntarism will be affected by that person's development in terms of cognitive abilities, emotional maturity, and moral character. In essence, a child is less capable of deliberate, voluntary choice than is an adolescent or an adult. The second domain of influence on the capacity for voluntarism is illness-related considerations, such as diminished concentration, poor energy, and indecisiveness (e.g., as seen in some people with major depression) and apathy, cognitive deficits, and ambivalence (e.g., as seen in some people with schizophrenia). These illness manifestations may vary, with multiple symptoms at some times and fewer symptoms at other times. Illness-related considerations can prevent the individual from collecting his thoughts, feelings, and personal values to make a coherent and enduring choice.

Third, psychological issues and cultural and religious values influence voluntarism. They may contribute in a manner that enhances the person's sense of individual autonomy and empowerment. Alternatively, these influences may diminish voluntarism or may simply render less relevant various factors associated with voluntarism. Even seeing one's ideal self as a separate, autonomous individual—as an agent able to decide and act—is a perspective that some have characterized as distinctly "Western," culture-bound, and masculine in its approach to decision making. Finally, external features and pressures are potent influences on voluntarism. For example, a nursing home resident may be so dependent upon her caregivers that she has little voice in a new treatment decision. Similarly, a patient who is admitted involuntarily to a psychiatric unit can, by law, refuse medication and other treatments but may feel coerced by his context to accept these interventions.

■ DIFFERING STANDARDS FOR CONSENT

Sometimes the most critical task for a clinician is to assess what kind of decision a person is truly capable of making—can the ill individual make *part* of the decision, select someone to make the decision, or identify someone to describe her values to help influence the ultimate decision? For instance, although a person with mild to moderate dementia may be incapable of making a choice about use of a new medication or a sophisticated imaging study, she may be capable of deciding which person knows her best and can best represent her views in making such a choice. One of us (LWR) commonly uses the point in teaching that although we may not be capable of making a decision to enter an elaborate clinical treatment regimen, we may well be capable of deciding who loves us and can be trusted to make that decision. It may also be possible to break down clinical decisions into component parts and to introduce each element incrementally to the patient, later pulling together the whole set in a manner that makes sense and is understandable. In other words, decisional capacity must be examined in relation to the nature of the decision. It may be that a different decision, or set of decisions, will be possible for a given individual.

In general, the stringency of the standard for consent or refusal of recommended treatment is driven by the level of risk and the overall risk–benefit ratio that accompany the choice (Figure 4–2) (Drane 1984). If acceptance of a recommended treatment has few and less serious risks, then the standard is relatively low. If, on the other hand, refusing a recommended treatment is likely to have many or more severe risks, the standard's stringency is relatively high. The rationale for this variation within the standard is not arbitrariness or paternalism, but rather follows the duty to faithfully act with beneficence and nonmaleficence as guideposts and to ensure that an illness-related condition is not interfering with the judgment of the patient who is making a choice that may put him or her in harm's way.

Emergency or Acute Care

To a large extent, the patient's clinical situation determines the standard for informed consent in emergent or acute care. In such situations, there may be little time for information sharing and mutual decision making. Acting beneficently—that is, with a view toward saving the life or preserving the health of the patient—is the clinician's duty in such circumstances. This action on behalf of the patient is held to be ethically and legally justifiable; it is presumed that in such emergency situations the patient wishes to be helped in the best manner known to the clinician and that the clinician has permission to act with the patient's well-being and best interests at heart. Often the patient, if alert and conscious, will explicitly assent to treatment in these circumstances (i.e., voluntarily accept the choice proffered by the clinician at the time). If the patient is unconscious or is unable to communicate at all, the clinician acts with the "implied consent" or "presumed consent" of the patient.

When the patient refuses treatment in an emergent situation, however, a very rigorous standard for consent must be applied, for

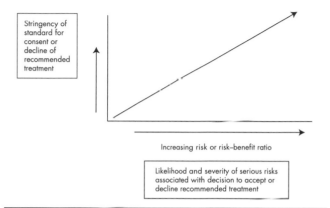

FIGURE 4–2. **The "sliding scale" of consent standards.**

two reasons: 1) the likelihood of an adverse outcome, and 2) the possibility that clinical factors may be adversely affecting the patient's judgment. Undiagnosed delirium, delusional thinking, severe physical pain, emotional distress, and interpersonal pressure all may undermine a patient's ability to make a fully informed, autonomous choice in an acute situation, as noted in the Appendix to this chapter. When a patient refuses treatment, focusing too much on the patient's philosophical and legal right to "self-determination" may obscure the presence of a significant clinical issue that requires attention. Clarification of underlying clinical considerations in such circumstances is the caregiver's primary responsibility, grounded in the bioethics principles of respect for persons, clinical standards of care, fidelity, and beneficence. The intention here is not to undermine the patient's autonomy, but rather to empower the clinician *only insofar as* to help advance the health and well-being of the patient and to ensure that the patient is optimally able to express his or her true wishes to accept or decline a given therapeutic approach.

In sum, in situations where clinical decisions may have very serious or irreversible health consequences, including death, informed refusal of treatment must fulfill the most stringent standards. These are the decisions that "fly in the face of both professional and public rationality." The clinician must be certain that medical and psychiatric issues are carefully assessed for their contribution to the patient's choice (e.g., insufficient pain treatment in a cancer patient requesting that life-saving treatment be discontinued). The patient must clearly demonstrate knowledge of, understanding of, and appreciation for the ramifications of the decision to refuse care. There must be an indication that this choice is consistent with his or her life patterns and personal values (e.g., decisions to refuse certain kinds of treatments in the past). External coercive forces (e.g., a family member that is pushing the patient to refuse care because of the family's religious beliefs or concern over financial problems) must be eliminated insofar as possible. In keeping with the duties of beneficence, fidelity, and clinical competence, seeking a "second chance" by keeping a patient alive and safe, to whatever extent possible, is essential in any situation in which the individual's wishes are unclear, inconsistent, or compromised by clinical symptoms.

Care for Chronic Illness

The goal of informed, voluntary decision making may be more clearly fulfilled in the context of care for chronic illness. Over the course of time, the clinician may come to know the patient—his symptoms, his values and concerns, his responsiveness to treatment interventions, and his personal supports. In turn, the patient may acquire a greater sense of trust, come to express himself with greater openness, and gather more complete information about the illness and potential therapeutic interventions over time. The patient with a chronic illness also lives out the consequences of side effects, adverse reactions, and benefits of treatments in a manner different from the patient with a time-limited health problem. In this context, the patient may better appreciate how his illness and treatment affect other aspects of his life, and it is possible for the clinician to come to know the patient's preferences and concerns with greater certainty. Expressing autonomous wishes and deciding on specific treatment approaches and the overall goals of therapy through mutual understanding and dialogue are intrinsically more possible in the context of chronic illness. Consequently, the standard for consent in chronic illness is very rigorous in terms of attempting to increase the patient's level of information, seeking opportunities to enhance decision making, and creating the circumstances in which patients may indicate their wishes and hopes.

As an illustration of how a consent discussion can facilitate the aims of the therapeutic relationship in chronic care, consider the example of a patient with recurrent, very severe depression who is unresponsive to medications and psychotherapy but who has previously experienced relatively rapid recovery with ECT. Clarification of outcomes associated with these dramatically different treatment approaches provides an occasion for the clinician to understand ethically relevant factors in the patient's treatment choices. The patient expresses interest in trying one of the newly released antidepressant medications but states that she is willing to undergo ECT again "if it will help more." With this patient, clarification of what the patient means by "helping more" is important. Does she mean "help with severity of symptoms right now," "help me to function while I'm waiting for the worst of the symptoms to go away," "help get rid of most of the symptoms as quickly as possible," or "help prevent future periods of depression"? Symptom severity, ability to "cope" while depressed, length of time until improvement, and prevention are quite different "outcome" dimensions in terms of the experience of the depressed patient, and different therapies may have different strengths in these various dimensions. An intensive course of ECT may help address very severe depressive symptoms quickly but may not facilitate social role functioning during the treatment period. Alternatively, psychosocial interventions may assist the patient who needs to perform critical work activities while waiting for antidepressant medications to bring about symptom improvement. A consent dialogue focused on outcomes thus allows for integration of clinical knowledge of potential treatments with the concerns, duties, and personal values of the patient.

Routine and Preventive Care

Routine or preventive care that is focused on the benefit of the patient and that presents little risk entails a less rigorous level of consent. Examples of such care include drawing a serum lithium level or performing thyroid and renal function tests. It is presumed that patients understand that such tests are clinically valuable and are associated with relatively few risks and harms. Clinicians should review the need for the information from these tests, but formal, detailed consent procedures are not necessary. Neuroimaging, HIV testing, and neuropsychiatric assessments, although common diagnostic procedures, represent greater biological and psychosocial risks to patients and, for this reason, require a more systematic and intensive approach to consent.

■ ADVANCE DIRECTIVES AND SURROGATE DECISION MAKING

Through advance directives, patients articulate their preferences for future care. Advance directives often are formal written papers created and signed by the patient; they may also consist of a body of documentation developed by the patient, family members, and clinicians to articulate his or her wishes and values regarding personal health care. Ideally, they will document the person's values and pattern of life choices as they relate to possible future decisions that are carefully described and envisioned. Advance directives are most helpful when they have ecological validity—that is, when they have enough depth and texture to be applied meaningfully. The bald statement, "I don't want machines," or "I don't want to be in the hospital," does not convey enough and can cause more harm than good in honoring an individual's stated preferences. Documents that characterize the thinking and the values shaping the stated choices, in light of multiple different scenarios, will be of greatest assistance to clinicians and families. Published materials such as "The Values History" and "The Five Wishes" are excellent tools for facilitating discussions of personal values and preferences with patients or within families with respect to many medical decisions, especially end-of-life care.

Advance directives are useful in several ways. First, they serve as a reference for the clinician if the patient becomes decisionally incapable or compromised. For example, knowing that he had a pattern of very compromised judgment during periods of mania, a patient with bipolar disorder completed an advance directive requesting that treatment be instituted despite his (anticipated) protests. Advance directives also provide evidence of the patient's past personal health care preferences that may result in controversial clinical decisions. For instance, advance directives may become critical when patients refuse treatment based on deeply and consistently held personal convictions (e.g., refusal of blood transfusions by a patient who is a Jehovah's Witness). Ideally, these issues will not be addressed for the first time in a moment of great crisis. They should be anticipated, discussed, and documented carefully beforehand.

Advance directives do not—ever—replace the wishes expressed by a patient who is currently decisionally capable. Moreover, there also should be opportunities to adapt, or even to reverse, earlier decisions, because one cannot always predict how one will feel in a crisis situation. For these reasons, advance directives may guide but should never supplant prudent, reflective clinical decision making.

In *surrogate decision making,* also referred to as *proxy* or *substitute decision making,* health care choices are made for the decisionally impaired patient by another person. This person may be a spouse, sibling, or adult child; a friend; or a court-appointed guardian. The surrogate decision maker has a large responsibility: he or she must serve the best interests and well-being of the patient ("best interests" standard) while seeking to make decisions that are faithful to the personal values and prior wishes of the patient ("substituted judgment" standard). Fulfilling this responsibility can be extremely difficult. In some situations, the best-interests and substituted-judgment standards do not yield the same result, in which case the person must abide by legal statutes operative in the state.

In other circumstances, the patient's values and wishes are not known. A patient may be too young or too cognitively compromised to have demonstrated personal values and wishes, for example. In yet other situations, the patient's values and wishes are known but conflict with the personal values and wishes of the surrogate decision maker—or, alternatively, with accepted standards of clinical care.

Consequently, in working with surrogate decision makers, it is important for clinicians to clarify the goals and values governing the choices made on behalf of the patient. It is also crucial that the patient's decisional capacity be assessed accurately and, in most circumstances, that the patient's symptoms be treated aggressively so that he or she can contribute to the choices made to whatever extent possible. In contrast with many medical situations, in which the patient's decisional ability diminishes over time, such efforts are especially important in the context of psychiatric illness, in which patients' decisional abilities may fluctuate.

■ EXAMPLES OF EMPIRICAL STUDIES RELATED TO CONSENT

Evidence gathered over the past four decades suggests that informed consent is an ideal that is often difficult to achieve in clinical care, perhaps particularly with mentally ill populations (Sugarman et al. 1999). A full overview of the empirical literature on consent, which is expanding rapidly, is beyond the scope of this text. This said, a number of studies of psychotic, affective, and dementia disorders have shown that symptoms of mental illness may adversely influence information-based or more strictly cognitive aspects of consent. For example, in the MacArthur Treatment Competence Study (Appelbaum and Grisso 1995), the decisional abilities of patients with schizophrenia or major depression, patients with ischemic heart disease, and nonpatient community volunteers (total N=498) were assessed. When acutely ill, the psychiatric patients in this study had greater difficulties with decision making on several formal cognitive measures than did the medically ill patients and the community participants. The problems were more severe for individuals with psychotic symptoms than for depressed individuals. Clinical treatment led to significant improvement of these deficits, resulting in closer resemblances across the three groups assessed (Appelbaum and Grisso 1995). Stanley and Stanley (1987) compared the reasoning ability of elderly individuals with major depression ($n=45$) and dementia ($n=38$) with elderly control subjects ($n=20$). In this study, the cognitively impaired dementia patients and, to a lesser extent, the depressed patients had significant deficits on a number of decision-making items. Similarly, Marson et al. (1995) used a clinical vignette–based instrument to measure the level of competency exhibited in medical treatment decisions by individuals with dementia and healthy comparison subjects. The findings revealed that greater severity of cognitive impairment in dementia correlated with diminished ability to formulate logical reasons for treatment choice (i.e., addressing the "rational reasons" dimension of decisional capacity). Global measures of dementia severity such as the Mini-Mental State Exam were not predictive of clinical decision-making capacity (Marson et al. 1995).

Problems arise with informed consent in medically ill populations as well. In an early, elegant study of 200 cancer patients who had consented the previous day to chemotherapy, radiation therapy, or surgical interventions, the majority of patients (75%) reported that the explanations offered during the consent process had helped them to decide about their care. However, when questioned closely, only 60% actually understood the nature and purpose of the procedure. Only 55% could correctly identify a single risk of the proposed treatment to which they had consented (Cassileth et al. 1991). A survey study comparing breast cancer patients in clinical trials and healthy control subjects ($n=142$) showed that the cancer patients retained less, but, importantly, were provided with less information (e.g., written descriptions, expected physical discomforts, side effects) during the consent process of research protocols (Tomamichel et al. 1995). A study of 861 people living with HIV-related illness revealed that whereas all had clear wishes regarding their care, only 35.8% had spoken with their physician about their preferred care (Mouton et al. 1997). Barriers to informed consent identified in an observation and structured interview study on a surgical ward and a medical ward included patient and physician attitudes that minimized the importance of consent processes, the "general passivity" of inpatients and acutely ill individuals, the complexity of the medical system, and the sheer number of decisions that needed to be made during the course of a given patient's treatment (Lidz et al. 1983).

Studies of advance directives and surrogate decision making have important clinical implications. Numerous surveys and interview-based projects have revealed that advance directives are underutilized and that patient preferences are rarely identified prospectively (Bradley et al. 1998). In terms of surrogate decision making, several studies have shown that most elderly patients would prefer that a family member (e.g., a spouse or an adult child) serve as an alternative decision maker (High 1990). However, studies of hypothetical decision making by proxies suggest that such individuals may not assess patients' wishes accurately. Sachs et al. (1994) studied 42 decisionally capable dementia patients, 64 proxy decision makers, and 60 well elderly individuals and found that the decision makers' predictions of patient preferences were overall discordant with the patients' own stated wishes. Similarly, Warren et al. (1986) studied participation choices made by proxy decision makers and 168 decisionally capable nursing home patients with respect to hypothetical, minimal-risk research projects. The results demonstrated that the surrogate decision makers used criteria other than the patient's predicted preferences (e.g., attitudes toward research) in making these choices.

Nevertheless, evidence is emerging that the deficits and barriers that hamper the consent process for mentally and physically ill patients may be amenable to intervention. Interventions in which information is presented verbally and in writing, using clear and understandable language, have been shown to improve patients' understanding of consent decisions (Carpenter et al. 2000). The timing of consent information—for instance, providing information in a relaxed manner or on repeated occasions—is important to patients' abilities to integrate and apply these data (Wirshing et al. 1998). Treatment of symptoms, ranging from hallucinations to physical pain, has been observed to improve the quality of patients' decision making. Finally, clinician behaviors that demonstrate respect for and commitment to the consent process (e.g., devoting ample time to the consent dialogue) have been found to be valued by patients and surrogate decision makers (Roberts et al. 2000). The observation that educational efforts, symptom treatment, and attitudinal obstacles can be addressed suggests a number of constructive approaches to consent in the context of clinical care.

■ CONSTRUCTIVE APPROACHES TO THE PROCESS OF CONSENT

It has long been recognized that informed consent is not reducible to a piece of paper. A signature on even the most thoughtfully crafted consent form is meaningless if the patient was poorly informed, if he did not understand the choice at hand, or if his decision was coerced. Informed consent is thus a process that hinges on the clinician's professional integrity and attunement. It requires sensitivity. It entails dialogue. It takes time. It involves posing the right questions for consideration. There are several constructive steps clinicians may take to support the process of consent.

A sound informed-consent process requires that clinicians closely attend to relationship, information sharing, decision-making abilities, and voluntarism issues (Table 4–1). The process of imparting consent information, for instance, requires attention to the patient's interpersonal cues and communication style. The information should be "pitched" to the correct educational level and optimally will incorporate both verbal and written materials. Moreover, the process requires a sense of timing and context so that patients can absorb the information they will need to make the choices they must without feeling confused or overwhelmed with facts that have no real personal relevance.

TABLE 4–1.   **Strategies for enhancing the effectiveness of informed-consent interactions**

1. **Information sharing**
   - Pay attention to the patient's interpersonal cues and communication style
   - Avoid technical jargon and provide information at the right level to foster understanding
   - Involve translators if necessary
   - Offer both verbal and written material whenever possible
   - Be aware of timing and context of information sharing so that patients do not experience an "information overload" devoid of personal meaning
   - Encourage the patient to seek advice from loved ones
   - Create opportunities for questions and dialogue

2. **Decisional capacity**
   - Assess the patient for deficits in decisional capacity
   - Provide emotional support and reassurance
   - For patients with decisional capacity deficits, approach things in a stepwise fashion—seek consent for beginning treatment and as the patient's symptoms and functioning improves, approach the patient for the larger decisions
   - If the patient is not capable of providing consent at all, use an appropriate family member as a designated alternative decision maker

3. **Voluntarism**
   - Establish a trusting relationship
   - Seek to understand the values and choices of the patient now and in the past
   - Address symptoms and illness phenomena (e.g., negative cognitive distortions, compromised insight) to whatever extent possible
   - Avoid pressuring the patient for a quick decision unless absolutely necessary; reduce pressures in the environment when possible

With respect to decisional capacity, the process of informed consent should enhance the patient's ability to make choices to whatever extent possible. Involvement of patient advocates, family members, or social workers and case managers and use of medications, supportive therapy, partial hospitalization, and other interventions may help to provide emotional support and to diminish illness symptoms so that patients are able to make the necessary decisions. Use of written documents such as advance directives, a Values instrument (see Appendix B: Values History Form in Chapter 11), and "The Five Wishes" can help encourage patients and families to talk about their health care preferences. It is also essential that the process of consent foster autonomy through repeated efforts to clarify the individual's wishes, past choices, relevant experiences, and symptoms. The process of exploring a patient's wishes can be very challenging, because psychological defenses and illness phenomena such as compromised insight may greatly influence the individual's ability to be fully autonomous. Similarly, prior experiences of involuntary treatment may profoundly undermine the patient's sense of self-efficacy and interpersonal power. It is for these reasons that trust and attunement in the clinician–patient relationship are essential to the informed consent process.

Case Scenarios

A 68-year-old woman with early Alzheimer's disease is asked to consent to treatment for acute pneumonia.

A 9-year-old child wishes to stop taking medications prescribed for his tic disorder because "other kids don't take pills at school."

A 56-year-old man with major depression with psychotic features initially rejects electroconvulsive therapy and then refuses antipsychotic treatment because he does not like the side effects of the medication.

A woman with bipolar disorder must ask permission of the leader of her religious community before she can consent to treatment with mood stabilizers.

A 43-year-old man with a personality disorder and alcohol dependence asks his physician not to tell him "anything" about a recommended sigmoidoscopy, because he "trusts" the doctor and does not want to know "about the specifics."

■ REFERENCES

Appelbaum PS, Grisso T: Assessing patients' capacities to consent to treatment. N Engl J Med 319:1635–1638, 1988

Appelbaum PS, Grisso T: The MacArthur Treatment Competence Study I, II, III. Law and Human Behavior 19(2):105–174, 1995

Bradley EH, Peiris V, Wetle T: Discussions about end-of-life care in nursing homes. J Am Geriatr Soc 46:1235–1241, 1998

Carpenter WT Jr, Gold JM, Lahti HC, et al: Decisional capacity for informed consent in schizophrenia research [see comments]. Arch Gen Psychiatry 57:533–538, 2000

Cassileth BR, Lusk EJ, Guerry D, et al: Survival and quality of life among patients receiving unproven as compared with conventional cancer therapy. N Engl J Med 324:1180–1185, 1991

Drane JF: Competency to give an informed consent. A model for making clinical assessments. JAMA 252:925–927, 1984

Ganzini L, Lee MA, Heintz RT, et al: The effect of depression treatment on elderly patients' preferences for life-sustaining medical therapy. Am J Psychiatry 151:1631–1636, 1994

High DM: Who will make health care decisions for me when I can't? J Aging Health 2(3):291–309, 1990

Lidz CW, Meisel A, Osterweis M, et al: Barriers to informed consent. Ann Intern Med 99:539–543, 1983

Marson DC, Ingram KK, Cody HA, et al: Assessing the competency of patients with Alzheimer's disease under different legal standards. A prototype instrument [see comments]. Arch Neurol 52:949–954, 1995

Mouton C, Teno JM, Mor V, et al: Communication of preferences for care among human immunodeficiency virus–infected patients. Barriers to informed decisions? Arch Fam Med 6:342–347, 1997

Roberts LW: Informed consent and the capacity for voluntarism. Am J Psychiatry 159:705–712, 2002

Roberts LW, Warner TD, Brody JL: Perspectives of patients with schizophrenia and psychiatrists regarding ethically important aspects of research participation. Am J Psychiatry 157:67–74, 2000

Sachs GA, Stocking CB, Stern R, et al: Ethical aspects of dementia research: informed consent and proxy consent. Clin Res 42:403–412, 1994

Stanley B, Stanley M: Psychiatric patients' comprehension of consent information. Psychopharmacol Bull 23:375–378, 1987

Sugarman J, McCrory DC, Powell D, et al: Empirical research on informed consent. An annotated bibliography [see comments]. Hastings Cent Rep 29(1):S1–S42, 1999

Tomamichel M, Sessa C, Herzig S, et al: Informed consent for phase I studies: evaluation of quantity and quality of information provided to patients. Ann Oncol 6(4):363–369, 1995

Warren JW, Sobal J, Tenney JH, et al: Informed consent by proxy. An issue in research with elderly patients. N Engl J Med 315:1124–1128, 1986

Wirshing DA, Wirshing WC, Marder SR, et al: Informed consent: assessment of comprehension. Am J Psychiatry 155:1508–1511, 1998

Appendix

CASES FOR DISCUSSION

■ CASE 1

A patient diagnosed with schizoaffective disorder was found wandering near his home and then was brought to a psychiatric crisis unit by police. It was discovered that he had superglued his eyelids shut, and it was imperative that he receive medical attention immediately. He was calm, would not speak, answered questions through nodding, writing, and hand gestures, but actively refused to get into an ambulance to be taken to the medical emergency room.

The clinician on duty that evening knew the patient well and was able to deduce that the patient's peculiar behavior was linked to a recurrent delusion he experienced when entering a manic period. In this case, the patient's ability to make a fully informed decision was impaired by his delusional belief that if people were to look into his eyes, or if he were to look at people, they would be instantly destroyed by powerful lasers that had been implanted there. He also believed that if he spoke of this "secret," he would be murdered by the forces that had implanted the lasers. Once the clinician initiated a conversation about these beliefs with the patient, it was possible to clarify that the patient wanted help and that he was willing to accept treatment but was terrified that he would hurt people or himself be killed.

The patient thus had some decisional ability and could offer assent for emergency care. Nevertheless, the clinical team also sought a legal process that would provide the involvement of a time-limited treatment guardian because of the patient's compromised insight and judgment and the specific content of his delusional material.

■ CASE 2

A patient demanded discharge 2 days after an emergency appendectomy. He was febrile, tachycardic, had signs of peritonitis, and yet
was insistent that he leave the hospital. The medical team was conflicted about granting the patient an "AMA [against medical advice]
discharge": the nurses and residents believed this to be the patient's
"right to refuse treatment," but the attending clinician did not agree.

In the initial psychiatric evaluation, the patient showed irritability, very subtle indications of diminished attention, was oriented
except to day of the week, and had no other apparent abnormalities
on an abbreviated mental status examination. He was noted to be
very tremulous. Within an hour, the patient was frankly agitated,
disoriented, and expressed disorganized thoughts. Additional history was then obtained in which it was revealed that the patient had
been drinking 1–2 pints of vodka daily prior to admission. Postsur-
gical infection in combination with alcohol withdrawal had trig-
gered a significant delirium, an early indication of which was his
treatment refusal and discharge demand. The patient's most dis-
tressing symptoms and disorientation resolved rapidly with treatment, and he withdrew his request to leave the hospital.

ETHICAL USE OF POWER IN HIGH-RISK SITUATIONS

Provision of mental health care involves ethical use of power—power that exists within the healing relationship and power that is entrusted to clinicians by society. Power, as we shall describe, is directly proportionate to the vulnerability and the emotional and physical risk present in a situation. The *ethical* use of power, on the other hand, is a fairly elusive concept. It is characterized by the intent (i.e., seeking to do good and to minimize harm to individuals and affected others) and by the outcome (i.e., whether it has in fact minimized suffering, preserved life, assured safety, or enhanced well-being) of the clinician's actions. Ethical use of power is expressed in diverse ways, ranging from offering a subtle interpretation in the course of intensive psychotherapy with a traumatized person to administering emergency medications and committing a seriously mentally ill person involuntarily to treatment on a locked psychiatric ward. Both actions may be undertaken with integrity and with faithful intent to help a suffering person and to protect others from harm—or not. And both actions may result in good outcomes for individuals and for affected members of society—or not—irrespective of original intent.

We begin this chapter with a brief discussion of the special ethical nature of the therapeutic relationship and the ethical use of power in different therapeutic activities inherent to mental health care. We then describe imperatives and safeguards in the use of power in high-risk situations (e.g., dangerous, suicidal, homicidal risk) and in ethically complex situations that may precipitate the specific therapeutic uses of power (e.g., treatment refusal by ill or decisionally compromised individuals). Many of these issues are also addressed in other chapters, such as in discussions of the therapeutic relationship (Chapter 3) and of informed consent (Chapter 4). In concluding, we offer suggestions for the ethical use of power in mental health care.

■ POWER AND VULNERABILITY IN THERAPEUTIC WORK

Central to the field of mental health care is the power to heal. This power derives from the strengths of the patient and the expertise of the clinician. With special training, knowledge, and experience, the clinician is able to alleviate, or at times lift completely, the burden of suffering associated with mental illness. Patients and families know that it is the psychiatrist, for example, who can prescribe potent medications to manage symptoms, offer reassurance, arrange hospitalization for safety and stabilization, and mobilize beneficial services. Interestingly, the power to heal in therapeutic work also derives from the interpersonal process between patient and clinician, which can be among the most intimate of all human relationships. In the context of psychotherapeutic work, patients share their life stories, their innermost concerns, their disquieting fantasies and fears, and their loves and losses with their caregivers. This openness and transparency make patients vulnerable, thus testing the limits of trust and interpersonal reliance.

It is the pairing of strength and vulnerability, trust and dependence that allows therapeutic healing to occur in the face of tragedy and serious suffering. However, this same vulnerability gives clinicians the power to harm, to reject, to misunderstand, or to exploit patients who struggle with the experience of mental illness, which itself may generate helplessness, despair, distress, and exceptional dependence on the clinician. For these reasons, it is incumbent upon the clinician to treat every interaction with the patient as having the potential to help or to harm and as being very significant in the life of the patient.

■ ETHICAL CONSIDERATIONS IN HIGH-RISK SITUATIONS

High-risk situations heighten the obligations of clinicians to use power responsibly to help ill individuals and to protect both them and others from harm. These are situations in which dangerous behavior, threats of suicide or homicide, or grave passive neglect due to mental illness become evident. Often, these situations are characterized by insufficient information; for instance, a seriously mentally ill patient with severe symptoms and erratic, impulsive behavior, who has recently arrived by bus from another town, is brought to the community mental health center for evaluation. Under such circumstances, it is possible for the clinician to make mistakes with serious consequences. For example, the clinician may underestimate the seriousness of a situation, thereby failing to intervene to protect the well-being and safety of the individual and others who are involved. On the other hand, it is also possible for the clinician to overinterpret and overreact to a situation, moving quickly to more aggressive interventions than may be necessary to fully discharge obligations to the patient and to society. Similarly, in addition to clinical assessment challenges in high-risk situations, judgment errors may occur in which clinicians overvalue independence and autonomy to the point of permitting decisionally compromised patients to take steps that are dangerous. Overvaluing of safety, however, may cause clinicians to usurp the rights of individuals who might be cared for adequately under less restrictive means. In a different scenario, clinicians who do not understand key issues at the interface of clinical medicine, ethics, and law or who do not recognize key countertransference issues may inadvertently shield individuals who are engaging in dangerous behavior not attributable to mental illness. This quiet, often unrecognized form of "collusion" may lead to diminished accountability of individuals and greater overall societal harm. In all of these cases, clinicians find themselves in binds, vulnerable to the risk of not adhering to appropriate standards for clinically and ethically sound care just as their patients are at risk for harms ranging from having their rights violated to losing their lives.

Consideration of these difficult issues inherent to high-risk situations reveals tensions across the competing values within our society. The profession of law, for instance, places primacy on autonomy and privacy, which translates in mental health care to "freedom from" involuntary commitment, treatment against one's will, overriding of confidentiality, or external control of finances. The profession of medicine, however, places primacy on the preservation of life, alleviation of suffering, and improved functioning and quality of everyday life. Clinicians thus may understand freedom as "freedom to" think clearly, to form relationships of care and concern, to not be overwhelmed by negative emotions or lack of emotion, to work meaningfully, and to enjoy simple pleasures. Legal imperatives in a high-risk situation may pertain to accountability in behavior, whereas ethical imperatives may relate more to explanations for behavior and to the sharing of responsibility in minimizing danger. Beyond these differences in emphasis of values shaping perspectives, duties, and decisions, there are differences in approaches to complexity: for example, whereas legal and political systems may engage in adversarial processes that rely on argument and debate, modern practices in mental health care and in clinical ethics may involve processes that seek common ground and consensus building. Both approaches are necessary to enable the mentally ill to receive treatment that is human *and* just, but in many high-risk situations societal imperatives may contradict each other.

■ SUICIDE, VIOLENT BEHAVIOR, AND MENTAL ILLNESS

Suicide represents a serious public health burden in our country, disproportionately affecting mentally ill persons. Suicide is consistently among the top 10 causes of death in the United States. In the past decade, hundreds of thousands of individuals have committed suicide, and literally millions have received emergency treatment for serious attempts. About 90% of those who commit suicide have a diagnosable mental disorder, most commonly depression, often complicated by comorbid substance abuse (National Institute of Mental Health 2001). Mentally ill ethnic minority youth, elderly white men, and other specific subgroups (e.g., indebted farmers) are at particularly high risk.

Unlike suicidality and mental illness, violent behavior and mental illness are not tightly linked (Anfang and Appelbaum 1996; Swanson et al. 1997). Findings of the Epidemiologic Catchment Area study indicate, for example, that 90% of persons with mental illness are nonviolent (Swanson et al. 1990). This study found that among violent individuals with mental illness, a feeling of being threatened or of losing internal control, agitation, substance abuse, and lack of treatment were all related to violent actions (Swanson et al. 1997). Other research has revealed that it is the presence not of delusions or hallucinations per se, but rather of command voices and beliefs that one is being controlled or threatened that precipitates violence in people with psychotic disorders (Harris and Rice 1997). One of the most poignant and publicized cases of such violence was the death of Kendra Webdale in 1999. Ms. Webdale was pushed under the wheels of an oncoming subway train by Andrew Goldstein, a patient with schizophrenia who had undergone multiple psychiatric admissions. Mr. Goldstein had been released after a 22-day hospitalization a few weeks before the murder. He told police that a spirit or ghost had entered his body and told him to push the young woman under a train. Reports at trial indicated that when taking medications, Mr. Goldstein was functional and nonviolent (Treatment Advocacy Center, Episodes Database). This incident provided much of the impetus for the passage of outpatient commitment laws in New York and other states.

Stories such as this one have *erroneously* convinced much of the public, and sadly some mental health professionals, that seriously mentally ill patients are likely to be violent. In a 1999 survey of 1,444 people by Link et al. (1999), 87% believed that violence was likely in an individual who showed symptoms of illegal drug abuse, 61% thought it likely in someone with schizophrenia, and 33% believed it likely in a person with depression. Two-thirds of respondents said they would use legal means to force people with substance abuse into treatment, and half reported that they would use similar interventions for treating people with schizophrenia. Ninety percent felt that those who were dangerous to themselves or others should be forcibly treated.

Ironically, the mentally ill are far more likely to be the victims of violent crime than the perpetrators. Hiday et al. (1999) investigated 331 involuntarily hospitalized psychiatric patients who were court-ordered to outpatient commitment after discharge. The rate of criminal victimization of these more seriously mentally ill individuals was two and a half times that of the general population. Interestingly, the patients' recognition of being vulnerable to crime was low—only 16.3% were concerned about their personal safety. Factors that contributed to victimization were substance use, urban dwelling, unstable housing, and personality disorder. A subsequent study demonstrated that outpatient commitment reduced the rate of criminal victimization, substance abuse, and violent incidents (Hiday et al. 2002b).

■ ETHICAL USE OF POWER IN SITUATIONS INVOLVING POTENTIAL FOR SELF-HARM AND HARM TO OTHERS

We wish to highlight four central ethical issues surrounding ethical use of power in relation to high-risk situations involving the potential for suicidal and violent behavior. Several issues to think through in dealing with these contexts are provided in Table 5–1.

Prediction

The first consideration pertains to the challenges of predicting suicidal and violent behavior. It is widely understood that accurate prediction of self-harm and violent behavior is extraordinarily difficult. With respect to suicide and parasuicidal behavior, one can be guided by past patterns of behavior and by a constellation of traditional risk factors as described above (e.g., male gender, being unmarried and without children) and risk factors newly recognized for

---

TABLE 5–1.   **Things to think through in high-risk situations**

- What clinical illness factors are driving the situation?
- What are the ethical and legal mandates governing the situation?
- What additional clinical information must you obtain to understand the situation more fully? What collateral sources of information (e.g., from medical records, family, police, others) have you reviewed?
- Who can you include in this decision-making process to double-check yourself, your facts, and your judgment?
- Does your patient agree with and accept the recommended treatment? Is the patient capable of this decision? Why or why not?
- What is the least intrusive, least restrictive intervention to assure the safety of the patient? An intended/threatened victim? The community at large?
- Have you documented your reasoning and the disposition of the case in terms of risk, your approach, and necessary treatment? Is it compliant with appropriate clinical and legal standards of care?

---

their potency (e.g., extreme anxiety, agitation, hopelessness) (Fawcett 2001). Hall and Platt (1999) reviewed risk factors for 100 patients who made severe suicide attempts. Factors predictive of suicidal behavior included severe anxiety; panic attacks; depressed mood; major affective disorder; loss of a relationship; recent alcohol or drug use; feelings of helplessness, hopelessness, and worthlessness; insomnia; anhedonia; inability to hold a job; and recent onset of impulsive behavior. Presence of a suicide note was not an accurate indicator in this study. In a comprehensive review of risk appraisal and management of violent behavior, Harris and Rice (1997) found that the factors most consistently associated with violence were male sex, youth, past antisocial and violent conduct, psychopathy, substance abuse, and aggression as a child. Major mental disorder or other psychiatric distress was a poor actuarial predictor of violence.

Thus, prediction of these high-risk behaviors is partly an issue of clinical acumen and awareness of patient risk factors, and it is certainly also a matter of curiosity, intuition, and diligence in evaluating patients, gathering additional data, and reviewing collateral materials. However, risk assessment is inherently probabilistic, which means that expertise will never fully eliminate uncertainty. This fact is cold comfort after an at-risk patient takes a self-harmful step or acts violently. For many reasons, ranging from ethical ideals to pragmatic parameters, one simply cannot hospitalize all individuals merely on the basis of risk of possible suicide or violence at some point in the future (Maltsberger 1994). Consequently, the clinician has the difficult task of balancing many complex factors in fulfilling the duty of caring for mentally ill individuals with the potential for enacting self-harmful and violent wishes and behaviors. Building appropriate safeguards is therefore critically important.

Duty to Intervene

The second consideration pertains to the professional obligation to intervene therapeutically in the context of severe illness. This obligation represents the confluence of a medical ethical duty to help and a legal duty to act to protect vulnerable or endangered members of society. The ethics concept related to this obligation is *beneficence*. The legal concept is *parens patriae*—literally translated as the "parental" responsibility to seek to keep an individual from harming him- or herself through active or passive means, invoking power of the state to act.

The duty to intervene therapeutically becomes ethically complex only when the ill individual wishes to decline care. In such situations, an intentional process to preserve the rights of the ill individual is enacted. This usually involves placing a patient on an "involuntary hold" for a time period specified by state law (e.g., 24 hours in some states, up to 7 days in others), during which the physician assumes responsibility for keeping the patient safe and administers only those treatments that are consented to by the patient or that are absolutely necessary to achieve this aim. This process seeks to ensure that the patient's autonomy is encroached upon only as much as is necessary to keep him or her safe and to allow for a formal determination of appropriate treatment in the context of a legal hearing.

Criteria for retaining a person against his or her wishes for reasons of mental illness fall under the jurisdiction of each state and, accordingly, may vary considerably. Such criteria ordinarily relate to two core elements, which must coexist: 1) *mental illness is present,* causing an individual to be *at risk for imminent harm to self and/or others,* by either *active or passive means;* and 2) the proposed intervention is *believed to be beneficial and effective* and is the *least restrictive means* of keeping the individual, or others, safe from harm. This set of criteria helps to prevent abuses of power, such as detaining a non–mentally ill person for inappropriate reasons or placing mentally ill individuals in more restrictive settings than is absolutely necessary. The emphasis on the "least restrictive means" has led to creation of the option of mandatory or involuntary *outpatient* commitment for treatment of some disorders, and this approach has met with initial success in the treatment of addiction and comorbidity. These criteria also help to distinguish duties to intervene for reasons of mental illness from duties to intervene for other reasons. For example, if a non–mentally ill person is purposely violent, society mandates that he or she should not be shielded by a mental health code, but rather should fall under the purview of the laws governing criminal behavior. The same is true for a mentally ill person who commits a violent act if it is determined that the mental illness was incidental to, not causal of, the behavior.

Empirical research on involuntary treatment has yielded interesting insights in regard to the ethical acceptability of such treatment. Some studies suggest, for example, that the experience of coercion is not related to efforts to persuade or the presence of incentives, but rather is associated with perceptions of threat, either physical or psychosocial in nature (Gardner et al. 1993). Lidz et al. (1995) found that patients who reported that they were listened to, validated, given a choice in the way in which the commitment was handled, and treated with dignity and justice had far fewer feelings of coercion despite the involuntary status. Schwartz et al. (1988) examined 24 involuntarily medicated patients; at discharge, 17 patients (70%) reported that their treatment refusal had been appropriately overridden and that they wished to be treated involuntarily again if a similar situation arose. Those who persisted in refusing treatment were highly grandiose, psychotic, and had not responded to intervention. Gardner et al. (1999) interviewed 433 inpatients about their involuntary hospitalization 2 days after admission and then again 4–8 weeks after discharge. Fifty-two percent revised their belief about not needing hospitalization, stating that in retrospect it was appropriate, whereas only 5% changed their views in the other direction. However, even those who reversed their decision in favor of hospitalization still regarded the hospitalization as coercive (Gardner et al. 1999). In addition, it appears that involuntary treatment may actually be beneficial, in addition to minimizing harm. A study by Swartz et al. (1999) compared 129 involuntarily hospitalized inpatients who received commitment to outpatient treatment with 135 such patients who were released. At 1-year follow-up, the patients assigned to outpatient commitment had 57% fewer admissions and 20 fewer hospital days. The intervention was particularly effective for patients with nonaffective psychosis, although its success depended on a high level of supervision. Empirical work has yet to be performed on newer approaches, such as psychiatric advance directives, to determine their effectiveness in minimizing the experience of coercion and enhancing the rights of mentally ill people.

Duty to Warn and Duty to Protect

The third consideration we wish to highlight pertains to confidentiality and the obligation to help others who may be in danger. These issues tragically collided in the *Tarasoff* case, described in Chapter 6. The 1974 and 1976 *Tarasoff* rulings in California changed the climate of psychiatric practice, mandating a duty both to warn and to protect individuals who are endangered by a potentially violent mentally ill person. In such situations, the patient's privilege of confidentiality is overridden by the imperative to seek to preserve others' safety (Anfang and Appelbaum 1996). The standard of care in these emergency situations is to inform the endangered individual of a threat and to try to assure his or her safety. It is also essential to obtain collateral information from police officers, family members, friends, or staff of other health care and social service agencies. Although clinicians clearly should make every effort to obtain the patient's permission for these contacts, if such permission is not granted, they must proceed to comply with their ethical and legal obligations.

A post-*Tarasoff* study found that 14% of psychiatrists in the United States had warned a third-party victim in the year preceding the survey. Forty-five percent of those who chose to report did so against their own best clinical judgment, and this figure was much higher than the percentage who had performed mandatory reporting for other reasons, such as child abuse (Givelber et al. 1984). The few studies that have investigated the impact of reporting on the therapeutic alliance have not substantiated the widespread concern that the ruling would have detrimental effects on the therapeutic relationship (Anfang and Appelbaum 1996). Of the 3,000 mental health professionals studied by Givelber et al. (1984), 70%–80% believed that an ethical duty to override confidentiality and to take action to protect a potential victim from a dangerous patient had existed prior to the *Tarasoff* rulings.

The duty to warn and protect has found an unexpected application in treating patients with HIV/AIDS who are engaging in unprotected sexual activity and who refuse to inform their sexual partners. The clinician's legal obligation varies by state, but the ethical conflicts and tensions inherent to this situation do not. Most ethical standards indicate that clinicians should make every effort to convince or assist the patient to inform his or her partners before they take action, either by reporting the behavior to the public health authorities or by themselves notifying the individuals at risk (American Psychiatric Association Commission on AIDS 1993).

Strengths and Accountability of Mentally Ill Persons

In discussions of power in the therapeutic relationship, it is natural to emphasize the potential vulnerability of the ill person. However, doing so may leave the impression that mentally ill people are so powerless and dependent that they have no responsibility for their own actions or treatment. Psychiatric patients often possess several overlapping vulnerabilities—such as minority status, poverty, gender, homelessness, lack of education, and medical illnesses—that expand and augment the power of psychiatrists, psychologists, physicians, and mental health caregivers in ways that are subtle, complex, and often culturally determined. On the other hand, mentally ill persons have equal rights and responsibilities in society, although they do have some additional protections as well. Furthermore, clinicians will attest to the heroic and virtuous individuals who, day in and day out, live through the reality of the most severe and devastating forms of mental illness. These individuals fully understand what it means to be responsible, to be good citizens, to be compassionate, and to endure a very unfair "deal" in life with great dignity. A paternalistic approach that further stigmatizes mentally ill people and inadvertently denies them equal human and moral standing in this world is fundamentally unjust and certainly unkind.

■ ETHICAL USE OF POWER AND TREATMENT REFUSAL

Mentally ill persons have an authentic right to refuse treatment. And they do. A 1990 study of refusal of antipsychotic medications over a 6-month period revealed that 103 of 1,434 hospitalized inpatients declined to accept their prescribed medications (Hoge et al. 1990). In this study, patients who refused medication tended to be older and of higher socioeconomic status than those who accepted medication; in regard to clinical features, the medication refusers had higher Brief Psychiatric Rating Scale scores and were less likely to have received medication for extrapyramidal side effects. Those who declined also had more negative attitudes toward hospitalization and treatment. Particularly worrisome was the finding that refusal was correlated with longer hospital stays and more frequent seclusion and restraint (Hoge et al. 1990).

Refusal of psychiatric treatment, particularly medication, has unique clinical and ethical aspects in comparison with treatment refusal in medical or surgical settings. The most important consideration is the decisional capacity of the patients, because this may be a direct manifestation of the illness process itself (Roth et al. 1982). When an elderly woman with depression rejects antidepressants, her refusal may well be an expression of the despair and negative cognitive distortions that are characteristic of this disorder. Empirical work suggests that denial (often of delusional proportions), mistrust, and thought disorder may be powerful inducers of treatment refusal (Appelbaum and Gutheil 1980; Marder et al. 1983). By current professional and clinical standards, the more grave the consequences of refusal, the more strongly the clinician is ethically required to override the patient's refusal. If, on the day of admission, a patient experiencing an exacerbation of posttraumatic stress disorder symptoms refuses to sit with his back to the door in a group meeting, it is probably not worth contesting. However, if a patient with schizophrenia admitted for chest pain after a cocaine binge will not allow an electrocardiogram because he believes he will be electrocuted, the clinician must address and frankly override the voiced objection.

Treatment refusal by a decisionally capable person who understands and appreciates the consequences of the decision and whose choice is shaped by deeply held and enduring personal values should simply be honored. Treatment refusal is not pathognomonic of decisional incapacity! (See Chapter 4.) This said, often simply listening to patients, allowing them to express their fears, and providing choices and reassurance may resolve the issue in a manner that is genuine. Enlisting family members, case managers, friends, or other nursing and support staff often can help address a patient's fears and objections (Simon 1992). Finally, attention to the very real and terrifying side effects of psychiatric treatment may be important in obtaining patients' authentic acceptance of treatment.

There will of course be times when all efforts to obtain consent for treatment fail, generally because the patient is too sick to have insight into the need for treatment. In these cases, clinicians must have recourse to whatever judicial options are available in their state and institution. Most states allow treatment on an emergency basis or permit expedited medication reviews, although locales vary in how strict the interpretation of an emergency is in terms of duration even in crises situations. When a patient is truly decisionally incapable and is not likely to regain this capacity without medication, a mental health court or judge can appoint a treatment guardian to act as a surrogate decision maker. Courts vary on whether they use a best-interest or substituted-judgment standard for the guardian. In cases where a surrogate decision maker has been court appointed, the adversarial nature of the court proceeding can be mitigated if the physician presents only the facts necessary to establish the case, treats the patient with respect and kindness, and makes every effort to explain to the patient that he or she is acting out of concern for the patient's well-being. On occasion, treatment guardians will not follow the medication recommendations of the treatment team, but clinicians can employ the same diplomatic techniques and interpersonal sensitivity used with patients in working toward a solution with the appointed guardian (Simon 1992).

■ ETHICAL USE OF COERCIVE PRESSURE IN MENTAL HEALTH CARE

It is widely accepted that intervention in the thoughts, feelings, relationships, and sometimes the liberties of mentally ill persons is a necessary part of their treatment because of the very nature of psychiatric disease. Ethical principles govern such intervention, such as seeking to help, to avoid harm, and to minimize encroachment on a person's personal rights. Intervention should never occur solely for the gratification or convenience of the clinician (Hiday et al. 2002a).

It is important to acknowledge differing perspectives on the issue of coercive pressure in mental health care. On one side of the debate are civil rights advocates, some consumer movements, and a number of psychiatrists such as Thomas Szasz (1976), who claim that any effort to treat a patient against his will is always coercion and inherently unethical. Proponents of this position disagree among themselves about whether violence toward self or others is a valid criterion for involuntary psychiatric admission or whether community sanctions and the criminal justice system should deal with these threats. Many of those who oppose involuntary commitment and forced treatment are protesting against the very real excesses of the past (when patients were warehoused for decades without due process) and of the present (in some countries, individuals are institutionalized on the "grounds" of mental illness merely because they hold nonconforming political beliefs). On the other side of the debate are patient organizations, such as the National Alliance for the Mentally Ill, and the majority of psychiatrists and physicians, who believe that schizophrenia, bipolar affective disorder, and depression are real neurobiological disorders that affect cognition and the expressed preferences of ill individuals. From this perspective, mental illness merits intensive treatment, as matters of beneficence and justice (National Alliance for the Mentally Ill 1987). Most proponents of commitment and forced treatment acknowledge the violation of rights that occurred in the past and the corresponding duty to protect the liberty of patients to the fullest extent possible. In all cases, these groups affirm that ill individuals must be treated with dignity and respect.

There is also, unfortunately, a darker side to the use of commitment, forced medication, restraint, and seclusion that is ethically unacceptable to all involved in this discussion: the abuse of power in treatment settings to demean or punish mentally ill individuals. In the rarest of cases, there may be sociopathic clinicians who seek out roles that place them in control of vulnerable individuals (Epstein and Simon 1990). More commonly, poorly screened and trained staff, or exhausted and demoralized clinicians, may inappropriately use their power against patients with chronic suicidality, personality disorders, psychopathy, or cognitive impairment. Clinicians who view treatment refusal as a challenge to their power may be more apt to react with anger. Realizing that the patient is expressing himself in one of the only ways left open to him in his virtually powerless situation can go a long way toward eliminating the physician's wish to punish or abandon a patient. In sum, the best clinicians will manage their own occasional feelings of antipathy toward patients through vigorous and honest self-scrutiny, teamwork, consultation, and proper self-care if they are to engage in ethical treatment of vulnerable mentally ill patients.

■ ENDEAVORING TO USE POWER ETHICALLY IN MENTAL HEALTH CARE

Ethical use of power in high-risk situations rests on several pillars. First, the principles of respect for persons, autonomy, beneficence, nonmaleficence, and justice together suggest the importance of economical and judicious use of power in high-risk situations. The clinician must act in a manner that involves the minimal exertion of power in achieving a necessary aim such as safety so that the mentally ill individual's rights are minimally encroached upon.

Second, mental health clinicians have complex obligations—therapeutically, ethically, and legally. Given these high stakes, clinicians in high-risk situations should never be completely "alone" in making tough decisions. They should seek consultation, gather advice from multidisciplinary colleagues, and intensively pursue additional information from multiple sources. They must be extraordinarily attentive to countertransference feelings and extraordinarily diligent in seeking, synthesizing, and documenting information and making clinical judgments. Knowledge of legal and policy requirements of the state and the setting is absolutely imperative. In the current care environment, legal and economic considerations too often determine clinical care. Clinicians who place the safety and well-being of patients and the community as their highest priority and who exemplify this advocacy in their therapeutic relationships are actually less likely than practitioners who are less cognizant of these issues to be the objects of legal actions or institutional censure (Hickson et al. 2002). This finding must be tempered by the humbling realities of the difficulty in predicting harmful behavior. These recommendations obviously cannot guarantee a beneficial clinical outcome, but they can help physicians to come away from even high-risk encounters with the conviction that they have exercised power ethically in the service of the patient and the community.

Third, making every effort to work with the patient therapeutically is essential (Table 5–2). Treating individuals with respect, compassion, and dignity; helping them to recognize their need for care and finding, together, acceptable and safe options; and integrating duties to report and to warn into the treatment interactions are all important strategies in this process. Many clinicians and ethicists have been concerned that they must assume a policelike or judicial role that is contrary to their mission as patient advocates and healers. Psychotherapists in particular may feel that the trust and confidentiality crucial to effect personal change may not be possible under current legal mandates and political pressure. For these reasons, individual clinicians must search their hearts and know their societally mandated and professionally affirmed duties to arrive at acceptable approaches to dealing with these complicated, multifaceted issues with their patients.

TABLE 5–2. **Working therapeutically in the ethical use of power**

- Understand treatment refusal as a possible expression of distress
- Ascertain the reasons for refusal
- Allow the patient to discuss his or her preferences and fears
- Explain the reason for the intervention in simple language
- Offer options for the disposition of treatment
- Appropriately enlist the assistance of family and friends
- Request support from nursing and support staff
- Assess decisional capacity and if necessary have recourse to the courts
- Attend to side effects—both long and short term, serious and bothersome
- Employ emergency treatment options where available
- Work to preserve the therapeutic alliance
- Utilize treatment guardians where appropriate

Case Scenarios

An unemployed man in a severe depressive episode voices the intent to kill his wife, children, and himself because he feels that they would all be "better off." He has a loaded gun in his closet.

A woman with postpartum psychosis has intrusive thoughts of harming her new baby.

An anorexic patient develops hypokalemia and cardiac arrhythmias but refuses hospitalization or intravenous nutrition.

A patient with posttraumatic disorder and alcohol dependence who made a serious suicide attempt 4 weeks ago is experiencing suicidal ideation and insomnia, but denies intent or plan to harm himself.

A bipolar patient fills out an advance directive stating that if he goes off lithium and relapses, he wants to be placed back on medication and hospitalized if necessary.

■ REFERENCES

American Psychiatric Association Commission on AIDS: Position statement on confidentiality, disclosure, and protection of others. Am J Psychiatry 150:852, 1993

Anfang SA, Appelbaum PS: Twenty years after *Tarasoff*: reviewing the duty to protect. Harv Rev Psychiatry 4(2):67–76, 1996

Appelbaum PS, Gutheil TG: Drug refusal: a study of psychiatric inpatients. Am J Psychiatry 137:340–346, 1980

Epstein RS, Simon RI: The Exploitation Index: an early warning indicator of boundary violations in psychotherapy. Bull Menninger Clin 54:450–465, 1990

Fawcett J: Treating impulsivity and anxiety in the suicidal patient. Ann N Y Acad Sci 932:94–102; discussion 102–105, 2001

Gardner W, Lidz CW, Hoge SK, et al: Patients' revisions of their beliefs about the need for hospitalization. Am J Psychiatry 156:1385–1391, 1999

Gardner W, Hoge SK, Bennett N, et al: Two scales for measuring patients' perceptions for coercion during mental hospital admission. Behav Sci Law 11(3):307–321, 1993

Givelber DJ, Bowers WJ, Blitch CL: Tarasoff, myth and reality: an empirical study of private law in action. Wisconsin Law Review 84(2):443–497, 1984

Hall RC, Platt DE: Suicide risk assessment: a review of risk factors for suicide in 100 patients who made severe suicide attempts. Evaluation of suicide risk in a time of managed care. Psychosomatics 40:18–27, 1999

Harris GT, Rice ME: Risk appraisal and management of violent behavior. Psychiatr Serv 48:1168–1176, 1997

Hickson GB, Federspiel CF, Pichert JW, et al: Patient complaints and malpractice risk. JAMA 287:2951–2957, 2002

Hiday VA, Swartz MS, Swanson JW, et al: Criminal victimization of persons with severe mental illness. Psychiatr Serv 50:62–68, 1999

Hiday VA, Swartz MS, Swanson JW, et al: Coercion in mental health care, in Ethics in Community Mental Health: Commonplace Concerns. Edited by Backlar P, Cutler DE. New York, Kluwer Academic, 2002a, pp 117–136

Hiday VA, Swartz MS, Swanson JW, et al: Impact of outpatient commitment on victimization of people with severe mental illness. Am J Psychiatry 159:1403–1411, 2002b

Hoge SK, Appelbaum PS, Lawlor T, et al: A prospective, multicenter study of patients' refusal of antipsychotic medication. Arch Gen Psychiatry 47:949–956, 1990

Lidz CW, Hoge SK, Gardner W, et al: Perceived coercion in mental hospital admission. Pressures and process. Arch Gen Psychiatry 52:1034–1039, 1995

Link BG, Phelan JC, Bresnahan M, et al: Public conceptions of mental illness: labels, causes, dangerousness, and social distance. Am J Public Health 89:1328–1333, 1999

Maltsberger JT: Calculated risks in the treatment of intractably suicidal patients. Psychiatry 57:199–212, 1994

Marder SR, Mebane A, Chien CP, et al: A comparison of patients who refuse and consent to neuroleptic treatment. Am J Psychiatry 140:470–472, 1983

National Alliance for the Mentally Ill: NAMI statement on involuntary outpatient commitment. Am Psychol 42:571–584, 1987

National Institute of Mental Health: In Harm's Way: Suicide in America (NIH Publ No. 03-4594). Bethesda, MD, National Institute of Mental Health, 2001

Roth LH, Appelbaum PS, Sallee R, et al: The dilemma of denial in the assessment of competency to refuse treatment. Am J Psychiatry 139:910–913, 1982

Schwartz HI, Vingiano W, Perez CB: Autonomy and the right to refuse treatment: patients' attitudes after involuntary medication. Hosp Community Psychiatry 39:1049–1054, 1988

Simon RI: Clinical Psychiatry and the Law, 2nd Edition. Washington, DC, American Psychiatric Press, 1992

Swanson J, Estroff S, Swartz M, et al: Violence and severe mental disorder in clinical and community populations: the effects of psychotic symptoms, comorbidity, and lack of treatment. Psychiatry 60:1–22, 1997

Swanson JW, Holzer CE 3rd, Ganju VK, et al: Violence and psychiatric disorder in the community: evidence from the Epidemiologic Catchment Area surveys. Hosp Community Psychiatry 41:761–770, 1990

Swartz MS, Swanson JW, Wagner HR, et al: Can involuntary outpatient commitment reduce hospital recidivism? Findings from a randomized trial with severely mentally ill individuals. Am J Psychiatry 156:1968–1975, 1999

Szasz TS: Involuntary psychiatry. University of Cincinnati Law Review 45(3):347–365, 1976

Treatment Advocacy Center: Episodes Database. Available at: http://www.psychlaws.org/ep.asp. Accessed August 31, 2002

6

CONFIDENTIALITY AND TRUTH TELLING

Clinicians acquire special knowledge about their patients and their colleagues. In the course of gathering personal histories, reviewing medical records, and performing physical evaluations, mental status examinations, and other assessments (e.g., HIV or genetic test results, psychological tests, imaging studies), clinicians are invited into the intimate lives of their patients. Similarly, clinicians are uniquely positioned to observe and evaluate the everyday professional practices of their colleagues as they respond to patient care situations that range from subtle to dramatic. With this special knowledge come two important professional ethics responsibilities: safeguarding confidentiality and truth telling.

Safeguarding patient *confidentiality* has been an enduring duty of physicians since the time of Hippocrates: "What I may see or hear in the course of treatment…in regard to the life of men…I will keep to myself, holding such things to be shameful to be spoken about" (Hippocratic Writings, *The Oath*). This duty derives from the broader philosophical concept of privacy—a notion that is highly valued in many cultures and that encompasses *nonintrusion, freedom to act without interference,* and *the safekeeping of personal information.* Protecting confidentiality is this third element of privacy and is simply defined as the duty not to disclose patient information without clear permission or in the absence of overriding legal imperatives.

Truth telling, the act of sharing one's knowledge and the limitations of one's knowledge with accuracy and with sensitivity to the clinical impact of the disclosure, is also an ethical imperative in medicine as practiced in this country. The truth-telling duty derives from the philosophical principle of respect for the truth (i.e., veracity). It entails that information be trustworthy and conveyed in a manner that can be understood and meaningfully applied by the patient. Beyond these responsibilities of individual clinicians, truth telling is an important principle in the structuring of health care systems to act honestly and to foster accurate disclosure of information (e.g., when medical mistakes occur or when decisions about covered services are being made). Deception, on the other hand, is the purposeful act of leading another individual to adopt a belief that one holds to be untrue, through either direct misinformation or incomplete information. Truth telling is especially important in speaking with patients about the unfortunate realities of their illnesses, about uncertainties and risks associated with treatment or research protocols, and about medical mistakes. Truth telling is thus at the heart of informed consent (see Chapter 4). Truth telling is also crucial for preservation of trust and integrity in the profession of medicine, resulting at times in therapeutic interventions with impaired colleagues and formal "whistle-blowing" efforts to prevent potential harm to patients or protocol participants. These aspects of the clinician's duty to tell the truth are reflected in the Preamble to the American Medical Association's *Code of Medical Ethics,* which states, "A physician shall uphold the standards of professionalism, be honest in all professional interactions, and strive to report physicians deficient in character or competence, or engaging in fraud or deception, to appropriate entities" (American Medical Association 2002–2003, principle II).

The tensions between confidentiality and truth-telling duties of clinicians often give rise to ethical dilemmas. The clinician who complies with mandatory reporting guidelines—for example, in situations of suspected child abuse—may fulfill her responsibility to "tell the truth" in her professional role but may also act against the patient's confidentiality wishes in the process. On the other hand, not disclosing a patient's diagnosis of HIV-related mania, encompassing sexual impulsivity and compromised judgment, to his spouse may be respectful of the patient's confidentiality preferences—and, in many states, the law—but may undermine the clinician's own sense that he or she has "dealt honestly" within the patient care situation. Documentation in the medical record, similarly, may be riddled with ethical problems. Clinicians may be tempted to omit or "tailor" patient information to achieve certain aims—for example, obscuring data that are embarrassing to the patient, framing patient information in a manner that facilitates insurance reimbursement, or minimizing mistakes that occur in patient care to protect against legal liability. Such practices violate ethical expectations within the medical professions but nevertheless occur. For these reasons, confidentiality and truth telling are linked, and clinical decision making often entails finding an ethically sound balance between these professional duties within the legal context of medical practice.

■ EXAMPLES OF EMPIRICAL STUDIES

In 1982, a study by Siegler, an internal medicine physician, found that roughly 75 health care personnel, including 6 attending physicians, 20 nurses, 15 students, 12 residents, 4 financial officers, 4 hospital reviewers, and others, legitimately had access to the chart of one patient during the course of a single, brief hospital stay (Siegler 1982). The exasperated patient remarked, "Perhaps you should tell me just what you people mean by 'confidentiality'!" In this day of managed systems of clinical care, with computerized medical charts, laboratory reports, and billing procedures and broad-scale sharing of data for research, it would be nearly impossible to develop an accurate estimate of the vast number of individuals with potential access to an individual patient's clinical records.

Empirical work in the area of confidentiality is very limited, but early findings suggest that efforts to protect patient confidentiality are variable and success difficult to achieve. In a self-report, structured interview study with 747 adolescents, 76% indicated that their confidentiality had been violated by a clinician in the past (Cogswell 1985). Female participants in this study identified confidentiality breaches far more often than did their male peers, especially in regard to reproductive health issues (72%) as opposed to general health issues (28%). In a novel study examining the actual behaviors of health professionals, inappropriate disclosures of patient information were noted on 14% of 300 observed hospital elevator rides at one institution (Ubel et al. 1995). A questionnaire study with 177 patients, 109 house staff, and 53 medical students further revealed that patients expect greater levels of respect for patient confidentiality than actually are present in the training hospital setting (Weiss 1982). For example, whereas only 17% of patients thought that it was common practice for medical personnel to talk with their spouses or partners about patient cases, 51% of house officers and 70% of students reported this perception. Only 9% of patients thought that clinicians would talk about patients as "interesting stories" at parties; 45% of students and 36% of house officers, however, felt that this was common.

Significant problems related to confidentiality have been shown to exist with respect to mental health treatment specifically. Complaints regarding confidentiality are a common trigger for investigations and disciplinary actions by the ethics committees of the American Psychiatric Association and the American Psychological Association (Pope and Vetter 1992). Nine percent of psychiatric outpatients and 15% of psychological outpatients in two other studies indicated that their therapists had breached confidentiality in the past (Wettstein 1994). A series of studies on group therapists' attitudes and behaviors found that whereas three-quarters of group therapists affirmed the importance of confidentiality, only 32% instructed their group participants about appropriate safeguards for patient disclosures (Roback et al. 1996). More than half (54%) of 100 members of the American Group Psychotherapy Association randomly surveyed reported that confidentiality had been breached by group members at least once in their practices.

Studies of patients with mental illness have also shown that about half experience significant concern about confidentiality but only a small proportion are aware of confidentiality measures that exist for their protection, e.g., surrounding documentation of sexual health issues or substance abuse treatment (Lindenthal and Thomas 1982; Wettstein 1994). Such findings are especially ominous in view of the fact that fears of confidentiality breaches have been repeatedly shown to prevent patients from seeking or engaging fully in necessary mental health care (Roback et al. 1996; Roberts et al. 1999; Wettstein 1994). A survey of 76 psychiatric patients and 76 community members revealed, for example, that one-quarter to one-half felt that the risk of a psychiatrist divulging personal information had prevented them "to a great extent" or "to some extent" from seeking mental health treatment.

In general medical care, the clinical value of protecting sensitive patient information has also been demonstrated empirically. In a study of 56 adult women patients, 91% indicated that "security, trust, and confidentiality" were among the top five qualities desired in a physician being consulted for advice on sexual health matters (Metz and Seifert 1988). Participants in a survey of 102 self-identified gay, lesbian, and bisexual youth ages 18–23 years reported far greater willingness to discuss their sexual orientation, sexual health concerns, and sexually risky behaviors after receiving accurate information and reassurance about confidentiality safeguards related to their care (Allen et al. 1998). An anonymous survey of 1,295 high school students revealed that 25% would forgo necessary treatment if their parents "might find out" (Cheng et al. 1993). Such findings underscore the importance of confidentiality protections to the use of health services and the effectiveness of clinical assessment and treatment planning.

Relatively few empirical studies exist in the area of truth telling in clinical care. Accurate disclosure of medical mistakes is an area that has begun to receive tremendous attention, however (Institute of Medicine 2000; Rubin and Zoloth 2000). Until relatively recently, only a few case reports had entered the literature (Baylis 1973; Finkelstein 1974). In 1997, Sweet and Bernat surveyed 150 randomly selected medical students, house officers, and attending physicians regarding two vignettes in which an "error of commission" occurred (i.e., a physician medication error resulting in coma, seizures, and enduring pain and a physician medication error resulting in patient death) and one vignette in which an "error of omission" occurred (i.e., a referral physician's failure to diagnose a patient's cancer, leading to unnecessary paralysis). A majority of participants (95% and 79%) indicated that they would tell the patient or his family truthfully about the mistake in the first two scenarios, but only 19% indicated that they would report the error of the colleague in the third scenario. Given that preventable adverse medication errors occur in at least 2% of hospital admissions, the findings of this study are relevant and important for clinicians (Sweet and Bernat 1997).

In terms of truthfully delivering "bad news" such as a poor-prognosis diagnosis to patients, a structured interview study of 32 U.S. physicians related to care of the terminally ill revealed that only 47% would tell the patient his diagnosis explicitly, whereas 22% would "use a euphemism" and 31% would not tell the patient at all (Miyaji 1993). In a recent cross-cultural study, 200 elderly Los Angeles residents were surveyed regarding truth-telling issues in diagnosing and treating terminal illness. Korean American (47%) and Mexican American (65%) participants were much less likely than Anglo (87%) and African American (88%) participants to believe that a patient should be told the diagnosis of metastatic cancer, and strong cultural differences were also found in opinions regarding the role of families and the relative influence of clinicians in making end-of-life decisions (Blackhall et al. 2001). A study of 677 medical geneticists in 18 nations similarly revealed considerable variability in their responses regarding whether they would 1) disclose the diagnosis of XY genotype in a female gender patient, 2) indicate which parent carries a translocation causing Down syndrome, or 3) reveal a diagnosis of Huntington's disease or hemophilia A *against* the wishes of the patient who was tested (Wertz et al. 1990). Interestingly, ethical withholding information from patients was the top-ranked topic (75% of respondents) deserving more curricular attention in a study of 181 psychiatry residents at 10 training programs (Roberts et al. 1996).

Significant disagreement exists regarding standards for ethical disclosure of patient information even in situations in which reporting is mandatory. Indeed, one recent study showed that up to 75% of clinicians would elect not to report a case of suspected child abuse, despite the fact that this "omission" would be in violation of the law (Wettstein 1994). In terms of falsely presenting or with-holding information, a U.S. survey with 211 physician participants published in 1989 revealed that a majority were willing to misrepresent a screening test as a diagnostic test in order to obtain insurance reimbursement. One-third said that they would offer incomplete or misleading information to family members regarding a medical mistake resulting in the death of a patient. Only 25% indicated that they "never" employed deception of any kind in patient care, and 27% agreed with the statement that patients "expected" them to "utilize deception" for patient benefit (Novack et al. 1989). A mail survey of 510 Kansas family and general practitioners revealed that small community size was a critical problem affecting patient privacy and physician behaviors related to confidentiality and truth telling. These physicians' techniques to protect patient confidentiality included: speaking with office staff about confidentiality (88%), omitting details from the medical record (69%), charting the importance of confidentiality (46%), omitting details from insurance forms (37%), failing to notify public health officials (21%), and misrepresenting facts in the medical record (6%) or on insurance forms (5%) (Ullom-Minnich and Kallail 1993).

Finally, only limited data have been reported on the ethical imperative to tell the truth as it relates to "whistle blowing." For instance, case data published by the Office of Research Integrity within the U.S. Public Health Service revealed 986 allegations of research misconduct in the 5-year period 1993–1997 inclusively (Price 1998). In 1996, 3,653 disciplinary actions against physicians occurred due to alleged violations of law, ethics, or practice standards in the United States. Beyond such anecdotal reports, however, no data currently exist on *failure* to report unethical colleague behavior in either the research or the clinical domain.

■ CONFIDENTIALITY AND TRUTH-TELLING DILEMMAS

There are circumstances when the risks associated with nondisclosure of patient information in mental health care are very great and outweigh the individual's privilege of confidentiality. Reporting clinical findings becomes ethically and legally justified in situations where there is a serious and imminent threat of physical harm to an identifiable and specific person, where breaking the confidence is likely to do good and to prevent harm (e.g., protection of the intended victim), and where other efforts to address the situation have failed or are insufficient clinically or legally. This is the basis for mandatory reporting in relation to the diagnosis of communicable diseases, discovery of gunshot or other crime-related wounds, suspicion of child or dependent-elder abuse, and drivers who are dangerous due to serious mental illness, epilepsy, or other conditions. Such disclosures are viewed as imperative in light of the need to protect vulnerable individuals and/or society.

The landmark legal case of *Tarasoff v. Regents of the University of California, 1974 and 1976* serves as a dramatic illustration. In this tragic case, a young woman named Tatiana Tarasoff was murdered by a graduate student, Prosenjit Poddar, who stabbed and shot her and who during the course of psychiatric care had previously disclosed his intention to kill Ms. Tarasoff. Although Mr. Poddar's threats were taken seriously by the clinicians involved in his treatment, efforts to commit him involuntarily for inpatient psychiatric care and to retain him in outpatient treatment by the University of California failed. Although his attorneys had argued that he had diminished capacity due to mental illness, the Superior Court of Alameda County, California, found Mr. Poddar guilty of second-degree murder in 1974. This verdict was overturned as the result of errors made by the judge in instructing the jury. Mr. Poddar was subsequently allowed to return to India. Because of the immense controversy it caused, the case was re-reviewed by the California court system in 1976, leading indelibly to the clinician's legal "duty to protect" potential victims of threatened violence.

From an ethical perspective, the tension between the professional principles of autonomy (i.e., furthering the rights and beliefs of patients) and nonmaleficence and beneficence (i.e., ultimately protecting the well-being of individuals) was central to the *Tarasoff* case. With the *Tarasoff* legal decision, fulfilling the responsibility to protect innocent others and society at large in circumstances of life-endangering patients became the predominant and enduring ethical imperative. Indeed, forensic issues often are predominant in making confidentiality decisions in clinical care. Specifically, there are five situations in which there are significant legal precedents suggesting that it is justifiable to disclose a patient's personal information without explicit permission:

1. In a clinical emergency
2. In the context of involuntary commitment
3. When necessary to protect third parties
4. In compliance with statutory reporting requirements
5. When speaking with colleagues to develop multidisciplinary clinical care plans

Within these legal parameters, however, there are a number of ethical judgments that must be made. Consider, for instance, the case of a hospitalized delusional patient who expresses homicidal intent but without reference to a specific individual. The patient is under close supervision, has no violence history, and is accepting medication. Is there any immediate need to take action to curtail the liberties of the patient or to report him to local officials? How about if the psychiatrist knows that the patient has a long-standing paranoid belief about his next-door neighbor and has made threats toward him in the past—is this sufficient to warrant action? What if the patient then leaves the ward without the knowledge or permission of the staff? Consider a second example related to the timing of a mandated report of suspected child abuse. How much data gathering should the clinician engage in *before* complying with legal imperatives to disclose information to state or county agencies? Which member of the multidisciplinary treatment team should make the report? How should the process around reporting the situation be documented in the parent's and the child's medical charts?

Confidentiality issues arising in more mundane, everyday situations are also complex. Consider the multidisciplinary team treatment planning situation: patient information disclosed or discovered in the context of a therapeutic relationship may be discussed openly by members of a large clinical care team. Patient information is also commonly entered into a written medical record or computer database. Similarly, in teaching settings, it is essential that trainees obtain guidance from their supervisors regarding all significant patient care matters. What confidentiality protections exist in these discussions? Is every aspect of the patient's life history included? How should sensitive material (e.g., related to drug use, sexual behavior, violence history, or HIV status) be documented? What limitations are placed on access to the patient's chart or to the computer database? What if the patient is also a part-time employee at the clinic where she is receiving care, because her group insurance policy requires this? Other routine situations in which confidentiality decisions arise include elective patient consultations; disclosures of patient data to insurance reviewers, managed care companies, or legal agencies; and appropriate disguise of "protected" patient information in clinical presentations and scientific papers. These widely ranging situations are often very difficult and may create significant ethical binds for clinicians.

The Health Insurance Portability and Accountability Act (HIPAA), originally introduced in 1996 and scheduled to transition fully into practice by April 2004, offers additional protections for patients' personal medical records. According to the U.S. Department of Health and Human Services, the aim of this set of regulations was to increase confidentiality protections and to balance the privacy needs of individuals with societal needs, such as public health, medical research, and quality assurance efforts and greater accountability around health care fraud and abuse. Key features of HIPAA include limitations on the use of personal health information by agencies and institutions for reasons other than direct clinical care (e.g., restrictions on use of data for research purposes), increased access by patients to their personal health records, increased access to patient data by governmental entities under some circumstances, and strengthened rights of patients regarding explicit advanced consent procedures for the release of identifiable data.

■ RESPONDING TO CONFIDENTIALITY AND TRUTH-TELLING DILEMMAS

Respect for individuals and their privacy, respect for the truth, and respect for the law are three general principles that guide the resolution of these kinds of clinical ethics dilemmas. Although the three principles may be in tension, as noted in the illustrations above, they often are congruent or can be combined harmoniously within the context of the therapeutic relationship of the patient. For example, when assessment of a family reveals evidence of emotional, physical, or sexual abuse of a child, mandatory reporting can be integrated constructively into the therapy by 1) informing the parents of the clinician's responsibility to protect the child, including the legal duty to notify authorities about the situation; 2) clarifying what the possible consequences of report may be and addressing the parents' fears; 3) inviting the parents to take responsibility for immediately reporting the situation in the presence of, and with support from, the clinician; 4) mobilizing additional clinical services to help the family cope in the crisis situation; and 5) offering reassurance that the family will not be abandoned by the caregivers. Through such efforts, it is possible to act therapeutically and to embody respect for individuals, the truth, and the law.

In general, strategies for resolving difficult dilemmas related to confidentiality and truth telling are severalfold. First, it is critical to inform patients of confidentiality issues early in the therapeutic relationship and to explain how the professional and legal obligations of the clinician fit within this relationship. It is important to offer accurate explanations of confidentiality protections and their realistic limitations, given the clinical care context. It is helpful to foreshadow for the patient how specific consent will be sought for "voluntary" disclosures of personal information—for example, in family meetings or to insurance company reviewers. This is especially crucial in discussing potentially stigmatizing health issues, such as mental illness symptoms, sexual behaviors, genetic information, HIV risks, and substance use patterns. In this same conversation, it is possible to introduce the topic of disclosure practices that arise due to legal imperatives, such as when threatening, neglectful, or harmful behaviors fall under mandatory reporting laws. When dealing with health data that might affect insurance or employment status, it is also valuable to clarify the patient's understanding of the impact of disclosure and the clinician's responsibilities for documenting and reporting data revealed in the course of clinical care. With some very difficult patients who may purposely seek to pressure—or even intimidate—patients and staff, for instance in some drug treatment programs or inpatient units, this material may be introduced very naturally into larger discussions of behavioral expectations and consequences within the treatment setting.

Second, gathering additional information and guidance from supervisors and colleagues is important when one is dealing with novel or especially difficult ethical dilemmas related to confidentiality and truth telling. For example, a clinician taking care of a patient with newly emerging substance abuse problems and a high-stress job involving the safety of others (e.g., air traffic controllers, military personnel) may wish to speak with a specialist in the area of chemical dependence to discuss indicators of more serious symptoms, appropriate treatment-compliance strategies, and professional obligations in the specific clinical context. In addition, to fulfill basic standards of care in this country, it is essential for all clinicians to provide patients with complete and timely information about their diagnoses, prognoses, and potential therapeutic options, including the option of no treatment at all. Any deviation from this "truth telling" ethics practice expectation requires careful justification, reflection, and documentation and should be undertaken only after consultation with knowledgeable colleagues.

Third, it is important for clinicians to think carefully about who has access to patient data and how such information is shared. Legally, patients "own" their personal information, whereas the caregiver's institution owns the actual clinical chart or computerized record. As noted in Chapter 3, this position which has been maintained historically is being eroded by the existence of large databases, some of which contain genetic data in addition to general health data, and by recent softening of regulations. Many individuals legitimately have access to the chart or computerized record in the clinical institutional setting (e.g., for direct patient care or quality assurance reasons), and when insurance releases have been obtained, the numbers of individuals with access to detailed information about individual patients can be very high. In answering the question of who should see or receive information from a patient's medical record, the new HIPAA regulations will offer additional protections to patients when information is sought for reasons other than direct patient care.

Other ethically important issues arise when information is given to patients or legal guardians. In accordance with HIPAA regulations, the majority of states in this country have laws explicitly allowing patients and guardians to have direct access to the medical chart. Sharing of information with patients and families must be understood within a therapeutic framework, however. Under ideal circumstances, patients and family members should be observed and supported during the process of reviewing the record. Alternatively, many clinicians will choose to sit with the patient in order to summarize and interpret orally the often confusing, potentially disturbing entries in the chart. Because the clinic, hospital, or medical facility actually possesses the chart and is legally responsible for it, patients should not be allowed to remove the record from the immediate care site. For these reasons, whenever possible, a secure, supervised area should be provided for chart review in health care settings.

A fourth strategy in dealing with confidentiality and truth-telling dilemmas is adopting the practice of revealing *only* what is absolutely necessary in all interactions outside of the clinician–patient relationship. This is important in both voluntary and involuntary disclosures in which personal information is released to anyone other than the patient (e.g., family members, insurers). This is also important in gathering advice from clinical colleagues. In general, such information should not be shared with an employer, unless this is clearly arranged and formally consented to by the patient at the time of the evaluation *or* is subject to mandatory reporting laws (e.g., uncontrolled seizure disorder in school bus driver, suicidality in an airplane pilot with major depression). With very few exceptions, the chart and the data contained therein should never be given over as a whole or "carte blanche" to anyone outside of the clinical care team or appropriate medical facility personnel. This is true even in cases in which there are legal imperatives (e.g., caring for victims of criminal assault such as rape), because the chart often contains a wide range of personal material that is not germane to the situation and that may be damaging to the patient if released. For these reasons, in order to comply with the law while also affording maximal protection to the patient, the clinician may find it necessary to provide only portions of the charted data or to review the relevant material verbally with the outside reviewer. Even though it may be very burdensome, the clinician's ethical duty to protect patient information is not abdicated in such circumstances.

Fifth, it is important to look for ways to improve how patient information is dealt with in the clinical care setting and clinical system. Sensitizing health care staff to the complex issues surrounding patient privacy and offering constructive guidelines for the workplace are critically important interventions for ensuring patient confidentiality. Maintaining secure and appropriately detailed personal notes or perhaps "shadow" charts—with clear notations in the "main" clinical record, including reference to the existence of the parallel protected chart—is a reasonable solution that many clinicians may employ when caring for patients with stigmatizing illnesses. This practice may be prohibited in many settings. In all circumstances, the main clinical record must document all key information needed to care for the patient. The development and implementation of appropriate procedures to protect patient information contained on computerized databases serves as a second example. Simple measures that may be adopted by health care facilities include use of passwords and encrypted codes that are periodically revised. Limiting access to those portions of the database that contain potentially stigmatizing information is also crucial. Encouraging employees to position their monitors so that the data presented on their computer screens are not visible to passersby may also be helpful on an individual-user basis. Similarly, efforts to minimize clinical interactions in public areas, such as hallways and elevators, will help prevent inadvertent breaches of patient confidentiality.

Finally, when dealing with threatening, abusive, or neglectful patient behavior that falls under mandatory reporting laws (e.g., harm to a child or a dependent adult) or with colleague incompetence or impairment, it is ideal to set up a safe and supportive situation in which individuals may report their own behavior directly. Individuals who are ill, whose judgment is compromised, and whose behavior is actually or potentially dangerous will benefit from a process in which they assume responsibility and take the initiative to help themselves.

A wide range of approaches are available to clinicians in resolving subtler everyday patient care dilemmas related to confidentiality and truth telling (Roberts et al. 2002) (Table 6–1). From the perspectives of the law and of ethical practice standards, some of these approaches are good, and some are not so good. Purposefully inaccurate documentation of patient information on an insurance form, for example, is not an acceptable ethical solution to the problem of safeguarding patient privacy. Nevertheless, clinicians may choose, ethically, not to document their *speculations* about a specific patient care situation if they are in the process of gathering information and expertise that may help clarify the issues involved. In some cases, however, even this may be ethically problematic—for example, when legal imperatives relate to clinicians' best judgments in the absence of complete information, such as mandatory reporting of "suspicion of abuse." The duty to be law-abiding and the duty to be truthful, even about clinical impressions based partly on evidence and partly on intuition, compels the caregiver to explore the situation in order to substantiate or discard the hypothesis about the patient and then to act accordingly.

There is one interesting exception in which "deception" has been viewed by the profession of medicine as ethically acceptable: the publication of case studies in which identification of the patient would be possible unless certain historical "details" are obscured in the presentation. Although it is optimal to obtain prospective con-

TABLE 6–1. Eight do's and don'ts for protecting confidentiality

Confidentiality issue	Don't	Do
Patient information	Don't assure your patients that whatever they tell you is confidential.	Do provide accurate information to your patients about the "realities" of confidentiality in your clinical care situation.
Medical records	Don't assure your patients that the medical record—whether printed or electronic—is confidential.	Do explain that the purpose of the medical record is to be *read* so that optimal care may be given.
Stigmatizing conditions	Don't avoid discussing the difficult issues that surround stigmatizing disorders.	Do strategize explicitly with your patients about potential confidentiality problems.
"Tailoring" the chart	Don't use practices that violate legal and ethical standards.	Do consider how to reconcile accuracy and privacy in all forms of documentation.
Significant others	Don't talk to "significant others" without permission from the patient.	Do remember to inquire about patient's important relationships.
Law and professional standards	Don't break the law or violate professional standards in the process of respecting confidentiality.	Do actively work to change laws and policies regarding confidentiality you think are unethical.
Lifelong learning	Don't neglect your commitment to lifelong learning—including ethical and legal considerations in confidentiality.	Do continue to learn about professional aspects of medicine and share your knowledge with colleagues.

TABLE 6-1.	Eight do's and don'ts for protecting confidentiality *(continued)*	
Confidentiality issue	**Don't**	**Do**
Consultation	Don't feel that you must be "on your own" when confronting difficult confidentiality questions.	Do seek consultation and direction from other sources: books, articles, continuing medical education, web sites, ethics consultants, and ethics committees.

Source. Adapted from Roberts LW, Geppert C, Bailey R: "Ethics in Psychiatric Practice: Essential Ethics Skills, Informed Consent, the Therapeutic Relationship, and Confidentiality." *Journal of Psychiatric Practice* 8(5):290–305, 2002. Used with permission.

sent for writing up a case, this may not always be possible. In such situations, it is within the traditions of clinical medicine to present cases in a manner that disguises the patient appropriately. This does not give permission for all types of inaccuracies, however. In composing these case studies, it is incumbent upon clinicians to use a minimum of "false" information in protecting the patient's identity and to alter no fundamental features of the case such that the clinical teaching point is itself based on an inaccuracy. For example, one should not claim that an adult patient is a child in a published report in order to characterize a childhood syndrome. Similarly, one should not present "imagined" therapeutic processes and outcomes as factual when describing a novel patient care situation in a case report. However, stating that the patient grew up in "a small family in the Midwest" when he actually grew up in a large family in the Pacific Northwest, when these factors are not relevant to the clinical situation but can help protect the patient, is, in this special circumstance, viewed as ethically acceptable. When developing a publication of this type, authors ideally will seek advice and collaboration from others in making judgments about how much of the truth to reveal, how much to omit, and what kinds of purposefully inaccurate information to include so as to adequately disguise and protect the patient. In many circumstances, it may also be appropriate for the authors to acknowledge explicitly their efforts to guard the identity of the patient through such strategies in the published report. The fact that some information in the case study is altered must be noted for the editors at the time of submission, as well.

Case Scenarios

A 17-year-old has been in psychotherapy for 2 years. He has generally been doing well in school and at home, but continues to have irritable periods and occasional outbursts of anger that are frightening to him and to his family. His mother calls the therapist and wants to know, "What is going on with my son?"

A 22-year-old woman was physically assaulted by a stranger at a party. She is evaluated in an emergency room, and the physician becomes concerned about alcohol use and depressed mood as reported by the patient over the previous year. Her father, who holds a very high-ranking position within the community hospital, asks that the physician not document these concerns, or the circumstances of the assault, in the patient's chart.

An employer calls a community psychiatrist and verbally requests information about a worker's mental health and addiction history. The employer tells the clinician that he is entitled to this information because "the company pays" for the patient's insurance, and the patient "has to be in good health to do his job."

A 34-year-old mother of three small children sees a psychiatrist for panic attacks that began after she was in a car accident at age 17 years. She has been psychiatrically stable for years and requires only semiannual "checkups." At her most recent visit, she tearfully confides in her psychiatrist, "I'm worried about my temper with my kids. I feel like a terrible mother, and I can't keep myself from spanking them."

■ REFERENCES

Allen LB, Glicken AD, Beach RK, et al: Adolescent health care experience of gay, lesbian, and bisexual young adults. J Adolesc Health 23:212–220, 1998

American Medical Association Council on Ethical and Judicial Affairs: Code of Medical Ethics: Current Opinions With Annotations, 2002–2003 Edition. Chicago, IL, American Medical Association, 2002

Baylis P: Medical negligence. Trans Med Soc Lond 89:75–80, 1973

Blackhall LJ, Frank G, Murphy S, et al: Bioethics in a different tongue: the case of truth-telling. J Urban Health 78:59–71, 2001

Cheng TL, Savageau JA, Sattler AL, et al: Confidentiality in health care. A survey of knowledge, perceptions, and attitudes among high school students [see comments]. JAMA 269:1404–1407, 1993

Cogswell BE: Cultivating the trust of adolescent patients. Fam Med 17:254–258, 1985

Finkelstein L: The impostor: aspects of his development. Psychoanal Q 43:85–114, 1974

Hippocratic Writings. Translated by Chadwick J, Mann WN. New York, Penguin Books, 1950

Institute of Medicine, Committee on Quality of Health Care in America: To Err is Human: Building a Safer Health System. Edited by Kohn LT, Corrigan JM, Donaldson MS. Washington, DC, National Academy Press, 2000

Lindenthal JJ, Thomas CS: Psychiatrists, the public, and confidentiality. J Nerv Ment Dis 170:319–323, 1982

Metz ME, Seifert MH: Women's expectations of physicians in sexual health concerns. Fam Pract Res J 7:141–152, 1988

Miyaji N: The power of compassion: truth-telling among American doctors in the care of dying patients. Soc Sci Med 36:249–264, 1993

Novack DH, Detering BJ, Arnold R, et al: Physicians' attitudes toward using deception to resolve difficult ethical problems [see comments]. JAMA 261:2980–2985, 1989

Pope KS, Vetter VA: Ethical dilemmas encountered by members of the American Psychological Association: a national survey. Am Psychol 47:397–411, 1992

Price AR: Anonymity and pseudonymity in whistleblowing to the U.S. Office of Research Integrity. Acad Med 73:467–472, 1998

Roback HB, Moore RF, Bloch FS, et al: Confidentiality in group psychotherapy: empirical findings and the law. Int J Group Psychother 46:117–135, 1996

Roberts LW, McCarty T, Lyketsos C, et al: What and how psychiatry residents at ten training programs wish to learn ethics. Academic Psychiatry 20:131–143, 1996

Roberts LW, Battaglia J, Smithpeter M, et al: An office on main street: health care dilemmas in small communities. Hastings Cent Rep 29:28–37, 1999

Roberts LW, Geppert C, Bailey R: Ethics in psychiatric practice: essential ethics skills, informed consent, the therapeutic relationship, and confidentiality. Journal of Psychiatric Practice 8(5):290–305, 2002

Rubin SB, Zoloth L: Margin of Error: The Ethics of Mistakes in the Practice of Medicine. Hagerstown, MD, University Publishing Group, 2000

Siegler M: Confidentiality in medicine—a decrepit concept. N Engl J Med 307:1518–1521, 1982

Sweet MP, Bernat JL: A study of the ethical duty of physicians to disclose errors. J Clin Ethics 8:341–348, 1997

Ubel PA, Zell MM, Miller DJ, et al: Elevator talk: observational study of inappropriate comments in a public space. Am J Med 99:190–194, 1995

Ullom-Minnich PD, Kallail KJ: Physicians' strategies for safeguarding confidentiality: the influence of community and practice characteristics. J Fam Pract 37:445–448, 1993

Weiss BD: Confidentiality expectations of patients, physicians, and medical students. JAMA 247:2695–2697, 1982

Wertz DC, Fletcher JC, Mulvihill JJ: Medical geneticists confront ethical dilemmas: cross-cultural comparisons among 18 nations. Am J Hum Genet 46:1200–1213, 1990

Wettstein RM: Confidentiality, in American Psychiatric Press Review of Psychiatry, Vol 13. Edited by Oldham JM, Riba MB. Washington, DC, American Psychiatric Press, 1994, pp 343–364

CARING FOR CHILDREN

With Gerald Belitz, Ph.D.

Clinical work with emotionally disturbed children is demanding and complex. When ethical and legal regulations are added to the therapeutic mosaic, the work becomes even more challenging. Every state has statutes delineating children's legal rights; however, few professional codes focus on the delivery of services to children or families. Clinicians and researchers must familiarize themselves with all relevant laws and practice of care standards, examine their own values, and collaborate with colleagues to ensure that ethical and quality care is provided to children.

■ PROFESSIONAL COMPETENCE

Each professional code of ethics emphasizes the necessity of practicing within the scope of professional competency. Proficiency as a child clinician or researcher is attained through formal education, training, and supervision. Clinical competency requires a thorough understanding of developmental processes in the domains of cognitive, emotional, social, and moral development; impulse and behavior regulation; identity formation; and family systems. It further demands an understanding of childhood psychopathology, developmental disorders, and learning disorders.

Children and adolescents are legally defined as minors and consequently are not sanctioned as independent and autonomous members of the community. Instead, children have parents or guardians who are legally imbued with the authority to make decisions for them. Both case law and state statutes have confirmed the primacy of parents in the lives of their children. However, as Melton (1999) has noted, adults other than parents are important in the socialization and care of children. These other adults can include teachers, clergy, coaches, health care providers, neighbors, and social service workers. Also, families are now defined in a multitude of ways.

Because children function in multiple environments, clinicians are advised to adopt an ecological approach in their work with children and families. An ecological or contextual view incorporates an understanding of the many systems that influence children, including the nuclear and extended family, educational systems, churches and religious beliefs, community standards, and sociocultural variables such as culture, ethnicity, and socioeconomic status. Correspondingly, clinicians need to learn to communicate with the important adults in the child's life and to coordinate the child's care with other professionals and agencies. Clinicians usually deliver care to children as part of a multidisciplinary treatment team. This requires all providers not only to understand the scope of their own professional practices but also to recognize and respect the important contributions of the other team members.

Professional competence demands that child specialists examine their own attitudes about children and adolescents, marriage, families, and child-rearing practices. Such examination may precipitate an exploration of the professional's own childhood. Professional competence further demands self-awareness about one's motivations for working with children. Unless clinicians become conscious of these underlying processes, they are at risk of abusing their power with children and families. Therapists may act out fantasies of being the child's protector or ideal parent rather than focusing on the child's and family's needs and strengths (Koocher and Keith-Spiegel 1990). Professionals who have their own unresolved parent–child conflicts may unknowingly precipitate clashes between the child and family or develop a nontherapeutic alliance with either the child or the adult. Any behavior that undermines or devalues the child, parent or family is a misuse of power. Child specialists are obligated to use their assigned authority and power only in the service of advancing the well-being of their patients.

■ CLINICAL TREATMENT ISSUES

Psychiatric treatment with children presents unique challenges to the clinician (Table 7–1). Not only are there questions about consent, but the clinician must sort out the ambiguities associated with confidential information, parental access to the medical record, documentation about other family members, and defining treatment goals.

TABLE 7–1.   **Special issues in the ethical care of children**

Professional competence
Consent
Confidentiality
Documentation
Treatment goals

Consent

Parental consent or permission is generally required before children can receive medical or mental health interventions; however, existing state laws allow children and adolescents a degree of autonomy in consenting to their own psychotherapy and other types of treatments. In addition to recognizing emancipated minors, such as those who are married, in the armed services, or emancipated by the courts, many states recognize the rights of mature minors. A mature minor possesses the requisite cognitive ability and maturity to understand the meaning and consequences of the proposed treatment and is capable of providing informed consent. *The Guttmacher Report on Public Policy* reviewed state laws and noted that several states explicitly authorize minors to consent to health care associated with substance abuse, mental health, and sexual activity. None of these states mandate parental notification (Boonstra and Nash 2000). The decision to notify parents is made only when the health care provider determines that such notification is in the best interest of the minor. As summarized in the report, all 50 states and the District of Columbia allow minors to consent to testing for and treatment of sexually transmitted diseases, 44 states and the District of Columbia allow minors who abuse alcohol or drugs to receive confidential treatment, and 20 states and the District of Columbia permit minors to consent to outpatient mental health services.

New Mexico's Children's Code serves as an illustrative example. The regulation reads, "Any child shall have the right, with or without parental consent, to consent to and receive individual psychotherapy, group psychotherapy, guidance, counseling or other forms of verbal therapy that do not include any aversive stimuli or substantial deprivations" (New Mexico Statutes Annotated 1978, Section §32A-6-14 [1995]). This statute does not establish a minimum age for consent or require parental consent for verbal outpatient treatments. However, the law stipulates that guardian consent or involvement is necessary for all other interventions. Guardian consent is required before psychotropic medications, residential treatments, or aversive interventions can be initiated with minors younger than age 14 years. Psychotropic medications and aversive treatments can be administered to mature minors 14 years or older if the minor consents, but only after the guardian is notified. Mature minors can be voluntarily admitted to a residential treatment center only with the permission of their guardian.

Knowledge of state regulations does not eliminate ethical questions in the outpatient care of minors. Providers must use clinical judgment, knowledge of state laws, and professional guidelines to inform their decisions. Parental notification may be circumvented if the minor is approaching emancipation or if parental involvement is likely to be deleterious to the minor. Failure to notify or involve parents may alienate the guardian system and may make successful treatment more difficult. In most instances, parental or guardian contribution will facilitate more effective treatment. Parental awareness and support of treatment is preferable because minors live with their parents and families, or foster parents, and are dependent on these adults for their well-being. Amelioration of the child's symptoms often requires modifications in the parents' behaviors, and such modifications cannot be achieved without their participation. Also, access to the other systems in which the child functions may not be possible without parental permission.

Confidentiality

Only the individual who consents to treatment can authorize the release of confidential information to a third party. With children, the adult guardian who provided informed consent for the treatment has the privilege of sanctioning a release of information. Even when a state statute allows minors to consent to confidential alcohol, drug, or outpatient mental health treatment, minors may not possess the right to authorize the release of information to third parties other than their guardians. In many states, such as New Mexico, the laws require the guardian of a minor under the age of 14 years to permit information to be shared with third parties. Typically, minors can release their own confidential information if they have legally consented to their own treatment. Virtually every state allows health care providers to share information with other providers without explicit parental permission when that information is considered necessary for the continuity of the minor's treatment or is necessary to protect the minor or others against imminent harm or death. The 1976 *Tarasoff* decision, which detailed the duty of clinicians to protect identifiable third parties from harm, is applicable for clinical work with patients of all ages.

Questions regarding the protection of confidential material from parents are more complicated. Many states allow minors to receive confidential treatment for problems related to substance abuse and sexuality. Although 20 states allow mature minors to consent to outpatient mental health treatment, providers retain the right to notify the guardians when it is in the best interest of the minor. Furthermore, a guardian has the right to access his or her child's medical record, even when the minor legally consented to the treatment. Most states allow providers to withhold information from the guardians if its disclosure is considered to be harmful to the child. California law classifies a negative effect on the provider's relationship with the minor patient as a justification for denying parental access to confidential information (DeKraai and Sales 1991).

Regulations provide practice guidelines. They do not resolve the most difficult ethical quandary: When is it appropriate to share confidential information with a parent? The distilled answer: when such disclosure is in the best interest of the child. Of course, determining what is in the child's best interest is a complex process. Successful resolution of this question begins at the initiation of treatment, when the clinician communicates the standards pertaining to confidentiality. This discussion, conducted in a manner congruent with the child's age and developmental level, identifies the particulars of sharing information with parents. At this point, the clinician clarifies whether the patient is the child, the parents, or the family and specifies the professional's relationship with each. As treatment progresses and the child matures, the guidelines concerning confidentiality may be modified.

Younger and more dependent children require a greater measure of parental involvement. Dilemmas usually occur with adolescents, who are struggling with autonomy and identity issues and who may be engaged in high-risk behaviors. It is respectful to explore with adolescents the process of sharing information with parents at the beginning of treatment and again when the need arises. More specifically, this decision to potentially share information with parents entails deciding whether the adolescent, the therapist, or both will communicate with the parent and the context in which information is shared.

When adolescents are apprised of the limits of confidentiality, they can make informed decisions about disclosing information to the therapist. Clinicians are advised to clearly convey their definition of high-risk behavior, dangerous situations, personal neglect, self-injury, and other circumstances that may warrant parental notification. Potential high-risk situations might include substance use, sexual activity, truancy, gang involvement, irresponsible driving behavior, extreme religious practices, unorthodox dieting practices, fascination with guns and other weapons, and illegal behaviors. Undoubtedly, every clinician has a list of dangerous scenarios that can trigger the process of communication with guardians. Central to the decision-making process is the clinician's understanding of the meaning of the specific behavior to the adolescent, the adolescent's view of the parent's capacity to emotionally support the child, and the family's cultural and religious beliefs. Also, mental health professionals need to understand their own feelings about their adolescent patients and their own moral principles in regard to the behaviors in question.

Problems related to documentation about family members are also common. Many parents release confidential information about their children without realizing that the medical record contains data about themselves or other family members. Clinicians are encouraged to educate parents about this potential release of private information. Possible options for preventing such unwanted disclosures include maintaining separate records on each family member, obtaining separate releases of information for each member, or deleting nonpatient material from the record before disclosing it to a third party. Many mental health providers are conscious of this possible exposure of private family information and are careful to document personal information only about the client.

Practice Dilemmas

Clinical work with children presents unique practice predicaments (Table 7–2). A survey of Minnesota psychologists noted several ethical problems associated with clinical boundaries: accepting hugs from clients, restraining out-of-control clients, giving food as a reward, accepting invitations to significant events, buying fund-raising items, giving gifts to clients, escorting clients to the restroom, and assisting preschoolers with toileting (Mannheim et al. 2002). The age of the child and the situational context were the key variables that influenced the respondents' ethical assessments of these behaviors. Generally, the clinician behaviors were viewed as more acceptable with younger children.

Boundary dilemmas about self-disclosures also exist. It is common for children to ask personal questions about the clinician,

TABLE 7–2. **Dilemmas in caring for children**

Clinical boundaries: giving and accepting gifts, restraining patients, using
  rewards, and accepting invitations to significant events in patients' lives
Self-disclosure about own childhood and children
Competing worldviews of child and parent regarding the clinical problem
  and treatment objectives
Reporting child abuse while trying to preserve the therapeutic alliance

ranging from, "Do you have children?" to "Did you use drugs when
you were a teenager?" Clinicians are advised to always maintain
their focus on the needs of their patients. It is important for providers to understand the questions within the context of the patients'
psychic world and the manner in which certain questions and patients affect them.

Competing worldviews held by the child and the parent represent another dilemma. This predicament is manifested early in treatment when the child disagrees with the parent's conception of the
problem and treatment objectives. A therapeutic alliance is difficult
to achieve if the youth perceives the clinician as an extension of the
parents. Effective and ethical treatment is contingent on actively engaging the child in the process of identifying the problems, developing a treatment plan, and establishing discharge criteria. Clinicians
are responsible for facilitating communication between the child and
parent and for mediating differing values and goals. When parents
maintain unusual beliefs that do not fit within larger societal norms,
clinicians may face very difficult dilemmas. For example, parents
may not believe in the use of medications, which may place the child
at unnecessary risk for serious, persistent, or life-threatening illness.
In such situations, the clinician should attempt to find common
ground but should ensure the safety of the child and seek to imple-
ment appropriate standards of clinical treatment. This duty to preserve the child's safety may, at times, entail the use of legal protections to protect the child's best interests and well-being.

Another critical question that has emerged pertains to the scar-
city of resources for mental health care for children. Barriers to care

may be concrete—such as the absence of mental health care services in certain rural and frontier regions of our country—or invisible and poorly identified—such as the obstacles to care for poor children, homeless children, recent immigrant children, or multiproblem, difficult-to-treat children. As an example, 25% of low-income children in our nation do not have any health care insurance (Annie E. Casey Foundation 2000).

This insufficiency of resources has been identified as a current health care crisis in our country (U.S. Department of Health and Human Services 2000). Two recent reports from the Surgeon General's Office estimate that 20% of children and adolescents have a mental disorder involving at least mild functional impairment and that up to 9% of children have serious impairment (U.S. Department of Health and Human Services 1999, 2000). Unfortunately, only one in five of these youths receive mental health treatment in any given year. The Surgeon General reports that an unnecessarily large number of children fail to have their emotional, behavioral, and developmental needs met because of the inadequacy of early intervention and treatment programs and the lack of an infrastructure dedicated to children's mental health services (U.S. Department of Health and Human Services 2000).

Protecting Children and Reporting Child Abuse

Mental health practitioners who care for children have special obligations to help protect children from harm. This translates to ensuring the safety of children who are self-harming or suicidal or who may be neglected or abused at home. These obligations guide treatment practices as well, in that they preclude the use of highly restrictive treatment procedures and severe discipline (e.g., inappropriate use of seclusion and restraint, purposely creating pain or discomfort in order to alter the behavior of a child). Every state has a statute requiring mental health professionals to report suspected child abuse to an identified state agency (DeKraai and Sales 1991). States impose penalties for failure to report and provide immunity from liability against good-faith reports. As a point of reference, nearly 3 million children are maltreated in our nation each year. The Administration on Children, Youth, and Families of the National Center on Child Abuse and Neglect reported a 98% increase in child maltreatment between 1986 and 1993. The report further concluded that increasing numbers of children are being seriously injured each year (Sedlak and Broadhurst 1996).

Ethical conflicts are most frequently connected to reports of child abuse. These reports challenge the principles of confidentiality and threaten the therapeutic relationship. Often, children and parents feel betrayed when a report is made, especially if the limits of confidentiality were not discussed at the beginning of treatment. Typically, the conflicts revolve around the questions of when and how to report. Determining what constitutes abuse is also difficult. Most states do not specifically define abuse or establish a threshold for suspicion. Local state agencies can provide examples of reportable abuse. Clinicians are counseled to explore their values and beliefs about corporal punishment, shouting, and other discipline styles before concluding a child is or is not being abused. The decision to report needs to be independent of the clinician's attitude about child protective service agencies and past experiences with reporting. However, the process of reporting may be affected by these variables.

There are a number of possible options for how to report; for example, the child or the parent may report, the clinician may report in the presence of the child or parent, the clinician may inform the child or parent either before or after the report, and the clinician may not inform the parent about the report. The decision of how to report is dependent on the provider's assessment of the psychological status of the child and parent and the parent's likely response to the report. The guiding principles are to act in the best interests of the child while complying with the law and using every clinical effort to maintain the therapeutic relationship with the child and the family.

■ RESEARCH

Individuals can participate in a research project if multiple safeguards are in place and informed consent is obtained. Legal precedent assumes that adults are competent to provide informed consent, while minors are not competent to provide their own consent. Significantly, the National Institutes of Health (1998) has established the goal of increasing the participation of children in research that investigates the treatment of disorders that affect children. How, then, do researchers include children in their studies?

Consent

The U.S. Department of Health and Human Services (DHHS) developed guidelines for conducting research with minors. Children are identified as a vulnerable population that requires safeguards to protect its rights and to prevent the undue risk of harm (U.S. Department of Health and Human Services 1983). Scholars point out that the minors who are recruited for studies possess vulnerabilities other than that of age. These youths are likely to have medical, psychiatric, or developmental disorders; to have school problems; or to be involved in juvenile justice or social service systems (Koocher and Keith-Spiegel 1990).

Parents and guardians are deemed to have the right to grant consent for their children. However, because consent can only be furnished by the individual participating in the research, parents can provide "permission" for their children's participation. DHHS guidelines require minors to assent to their own participation. This requirement translates to an affirmative agreement, with the absence of an objection representing an insufficient assent. Significantly, children can veto their own participation. Information about the research must be presented to the minor at a level commensurate to the child's age and developmental level. Indeed, children's capacity for assent is determined by their age, developmental maturity, and psychological state at the time of recruitment. Although children younger than 7 years are typically not considered to be capable of providing assent, younger children still have the right to learn about the research and to assent to their own involvement (Rosato 2000). Some empirical work suggests age 9 years as a "turning point" in cognition and voluntarism, allowing for greater ability to provide consent (Ondrusek et al. 1998). Recent research on capacity for consent and assent emphasizes the importance of noncognitive aspects of decision-making ability and of distinct coercive pressures that young people may experience (Roberts 2002).

Risk

The DHHS demarcated the safeguards that serve to protect minors from the potential harm associated with research. Risk is ascertained by evaluating the risk to the participant, the benefit to the participant, the benefit to similar children or to children in general, and the minor's capacity to provide assent. If the study exposes the child to no more than minimal risk, the minor's participation is acceptable with one parent's permission and the child's assent, irrespective of the possible benefit to the participant. Minimal risk is defined as posing risks no greater than those experienced in children's daily lives, assuming that daily life represents a safe and caring environment (Koocher and Keith-Spiegel 1990).

When the study presents more than minimal risk, minors can participate if the benefits are greater than the risks. The benefit to the participant must be at least equal to the potential benefit from the other treatments available to children with the same disorder. Participation can proceed if one parent grants permission and the child assents.

Research that exposes children to more than minimal risk and that offers no direct benefit to the participant can advance only if the study is likely to generate knowledge that will benefit children who are being treated for the same disorder as the participant. Furthermore, the minor must not endure any experiences that exceed in discomfort those sustained in a medical, dental, psychological, social, or educational situation (Rosato 2000). In these circumstances, permission of both parents, when applicable, and the assent of the minor are required.

Recent empirical work in this area emphasizes the importance of evaluating risk in relation to biological as well as psychosocial dimensions and from the perspective of the child, whose fears, physical discomfort, and expectations must be taken into consideration (Munir and Earls 1992).

Dilemmas

Current DHHS regulations do not recognize the concept of mature minors—that is, minors who are competent to provide their own consent. Competence is characterized by the ability to comprehend the relevant information, determine the benefit–risk ratio, and make a voluntary decision. A large body of research indicates that by age 14 years, most adolescents have developed the cognitive and social capacity to provide informed consent (Melton 1999; Rosato 2000). Interestingly, many states allow adolescents to consent to certain medical and mental health interventions and terminally ill adolescents to refuse life-sustaining care.

Many ethicists and scholars purport that the DHHS guidelines diminish the autonomy of mature minors (Melton 1999; Rosato 2000). Adolescents are regarded no differently from young children. Existing regulations do not allow an older adolescent to participate in a research protocol if the guardian refuses to grant permission. This regulation becomes an ethical dilemma when an adolescent assents to participate in research—because of its expected benefits either to him- or herself or to other adolescents with the same disorder—in the absence of parental permission.

Melton (1999) provided a thoughtful outline of mechanisms by which children and guardians can share the decision-making process. He proposed one model wherein children are afforded increased participation as they become developmentally more mature. He proposed another model in which guardians or other identified adults function as mentors or consultants for mature minors. In this model, the mature minor can provide consent.

An additional ethical consideration relates to a key societal justice issue that has been described as "scientific neglect" of vulnerable populations (Vitiello 2003). The vigorous self-advocacy of people with HIV infection and, to a lesser extent, of people with breast cancer has raised two important questions: First, does an individual have the "right" to access experimental research procedures, and second, do the health concerns of special populations, including elderly persons and children, receive adequate attention and resources? Within the field of psychiatry, the absence of adequate data on psychopharmacology in children has been identified as the provision of health care that is not evidence based, potentially causing unmeasured and unstudied harm (Martin et al. 2000). The off-label use of medications with children, which has significantly increased in recent years, represents even greater possibilities for harm. Rosato (2000) argued that children are being used as research subjects, without the benefit of a supervised and controlled study, when they are administered psychopharmacological agents that have not been approved for their age cohort or clinical diagnosis. Similarly, the paucity of systematic outcome data on children's mental health has left judges, social workers, teachers, and clinicians without information on the true impact of major decisions affecting children's lives (Jellinek et al. 1995).

■ CONCLUSIONS

Caring for mentally ill children and seeking to improve the understanding of children's illnesses and treatment through research involve clinical and ethical complexities that do not exist in work with adults (Table 7–3). Mental health practitioners who work with children must remain attentive to the vulnerability of their young patients. Moreover, these caregivers must have a broad repertoire of skills and abilities that allows them to assess, treat, and protect children; to advocate for them; and to work with families, agencies, and systems. They must also have the requisite courage and self-honesty for this ethically unique work. When ethical dilemmas like these arise in the care of children, it is valuable to remember the basic steps used in resolving clinical dilemmas—gathering more information, seeking consultation and advice, monitoring one's own motivations and actions, and maintaining an absolute commitment to preserving the physical and emotional safety of the child.

TABLE 7–3.   **Essential clinical and ethical skills of clinicians caring for children**

Remain attentive to the vulnerability of children and adolescents

Hone a broad repertoire of abilities to asses, treat, protect, and advocate for children

Develop skills to work with families, agencies, and systems

Strive for self-awareness and courage

Master information-gathering strategies to help resolve dilemmas

Seek consultation and advice

Monitor one's own actions and motivations

Maintain an absolute commitment to the safety and well-being of the patient

Case Scenarios

Psychotropic medication for a child with depression and attention-deficit disorder has the known risk of sudden cardiac death.

A 15-year-old runaway girl has just been the victim of a rape. She is terrified of the pelvic exam and other invasive aspects of the evaluation.

A 13-year-old boy in counseling for oppositional defiant disorder tells the counselor that he has experimented with alcohol and marijuana and but asks that his parents not be told.

In play therapy, a 7-year-old child who has been irritable and withdrawn begins to act out sexual behaviors. She becomes very distressed and tearful, and she appears frightened when it is time for her to return home with her mother and the mother's new boyfriend.

A 10-year-old girl being enrolled in a trial of new asthma medication is asked if she agrees with her parent's decision to have her participate in the trial. She becomes visibly distressed but says, "It's OK."

134

■ REFERENCES

Annie E. Casey Foundation: Kids Count data book. Baltimore, MD, Annie E. Casey Foundation, 2000

Boonstra H, Nash E: Minors and the right to consent to health care. The Guttmacher Report on Public Policy 3(4):4–8, 2000

DeKraai MB, Sales BD: Liability in child therapy and research. J Consult Clin Psychol 59:853–860, 1991

Jellinek MS, Little M, Benedict K, et al: Placement outcomes of 206 severely maltreated children in the Boston Juvenile Court system: a 7.5-year follow-up study. Child Abuse Negl 19:1051–1064, 1995

Koocher GP, Keith-Spiegel PC: Children, Ethics and the Law. Lincoln, NE, University of Nebraska Press, 1990

Mannheim CI, Sancilio M, Phipps-Yonas S, et al: Ethical ambiguities in the practice of child clinical psychology. Professional Psychology: Research and Practice 33:24–29, 2002

Martin A, Kaufman J, Charney D: Pharmacotherapy of early onset depression. Update and new directions. Child Adolesc Psychiatr Clin North Am 9:135–157, 2000

Melton GB: Parents and children: legal reform to facilitate children's participation. Am Psychol 54:935–944, 1999

Munir K, Earls F: Ethical principles governing research in child and adolescent psychiatry. J Am Acad Child Adolesc Psychiatry 31:408–414, 1992

National Institutes of Health: NIH Policy and Guidelines on the Inclusion of Children as Participants in Research Involving Human Subjects. Bethesda, MD, National Institutes of Health, 1998

New Mexico Statutes Annotated (NMSA) 1978; Chapter 32A Children's Code, Article 6 Children's Mental Health and Developmental Disabilities, §32A-6-14 Treatment and Habilitation of Children; Liability (1995)

Ondrusek N, Abramovich R, Pencharz P, et al: Empirical examination of the ability of children to consent to clinical research. J Med Ethics 24:158–165, 1998

Roberts LW: Informed consent and the capacity for voluntarism. Am J Psychiatry 159:705–712, 2002

Rosato J: The ethics of clinical trials: a child's view. J Law Med Ethics 28:362–378, 2000

Sedlak AJ, Broadhurst DD: Third National Incidence Study of Child Abuse and Neglect. Washington, DC, U.S. Department of Health and Human Services, Administration for Children and Families, Administration on Children, Youth and Families, National Center on Child Abuse and Neglect, 1996

U.S. Department of Health and Human Services: Code of Federal Regulations, Title 45: Public Welfare. Part 46: Protection of Human Subjects Regulation Governing Protections Afforded Children in Research (Subpart D). Washington, DC, U.S. Department of Health and Human Services, 1983

U.S. Department of Health and Human Services: Mental Health: A Report of the Surgeon General. Rockville, MD, U.S. Department of Health and Human Services, 1999

U.S. Department of Health and Human Services: Report of the Surgeon General's Conference on Children's Mental Health: A National Action Agenda. Washington, DC, U.S. Department of Health and Human Services, 2000

Vitiello B: Ethical considerations in psychopharmacological research involving children and adolescents. Psychopharmacology (Berl) 171:86–91, 2003

8

CARING FOR PEOPLE
WITH ADDICTIONS

With Michael Bogenschutz, M.D.

Addictions are best conceptualized as disorders similar to other chronic psychiatric and medical conditions (McLellan et al. 2000). Like their physical counterparts, addiction and comorbid disorders are prevalent and severe, and they lead to great suffering and societal burden. All of the major bioethics principles, including beneficence, fairness, respect for persons, and truth telling, apply to addictions (Table 8–1). Although the ethical issues that arise in addiction disorders are similar to those that arise in physical disorders, they differ in emphasis and in particulars. Ethical issues in addiction psychiatry, moreover, are made more complex by the role of stigma.

■ PREVALENCE AND SERIOUSNESS OF ADDICTION AND COMORBID DISORDERS

The DSM-IV-TR (American Psychiatric Association 2000) substance use disorders comprise abuse and dependence diagnoses for each major class of substance (alcohol, amphetamines, cannabis, cocaine, hallucinogens, inhalants, nicotine, opioids, phencyclidine, and sedative, hypnotic, or anxiolytic drugs). In the United States in 1999, an estimated 8.2 million people were dependent on alcohol, and 3.5 million were dependent on illicit drugs (National House-

---

TABLE 8–1.   **Ethical principles and issues in addiction**

Respect for persons—Stigma carries with it disrespect and discrimination, which are major considerations in the diagnosis and treatment intervention with addiction and comorbid disorders

Justice—Parity or equitable treatment for addiction and comorbid disorders represents the need for social justice in the allocation of resources for these conditions, which affect millions of people and pose a significant personal and societal burden

Personal responsibility and voluntarism—These are key concepts in addiction because of the fundamental nature of the illness and because addiction may involve use of substances that are unlawful to possess or use

Confidentiality—Special protections exist in relation to confidentiality and safeguarding privacy because of the risk of discrimination toward people who suffer from addictive disorders

Truth telling—Stigma and legal consequences of addictions may generate conflicts around truth telling for both patient and clinician

Therapeutic alliance—Because clinicians have access to substances that may be requested by patients with addictive disorders and because addictive disorders are characterized by periods of relapse, establishment of trust in the therapeutic alliance may be especially difficult

Nonmaleficence, or "do no harm"—Treatment of addiction requires a paradigm of seeking harm reduction through periods of remission or reduced use of addictive substances, as well as efforts to balance risks and benefits in minimizing the negative consequences of addiction

---

hold Survey on Drug Abuse 1999). Lifetime prevalence of alcohol use disorder is estimated at 13.5% to 23.5%. For drug use disorders, the lifetime prevalence is 6.1% to 11.9% (Kessler et al. 1994). Patients with substance use disorders have elevated rates of most psychiatric disorders—and, conversely, patients with most psychiatric disorders have elevated rates of substance use disorders. The overall odds ratio for co-occurrence of substance use disorders and other psychiatric disorders is 2.7, although comorbidity is much greater than this for certain disorders, such as schizophrenia, bipolar disorder, and antisocial personality disorder (Regier et al. 1993). The costs of substance use disorders, in terms of human suffering and economic impact, are staggering. People with substance use disorders die at markedly elevated rates. Overall mortality ratios (relative to the general population) are 2:1 for individuals with alcohol use disorders, 6:1 for opioid-dependent persons, and anywhere from 2:1 to 21:1 for persons with other drug use disorders. Ratios for unnatural death (suicide, homicide, and accidents) are substantially higher than those for total mortality, and such ratios tend to be particularly high in females (e.g., 18:1 for women with alcohol abuse or dependence relative to women in the general population) (Harris and Barraclough 1998). The total economic costs of substance use disorders in 1995 were estimated at $428.1 billion: $175.9 billion for alcohol, $138 billion for nicotine dependence, and $114.2 billion for other drugs (Rice et al. 1991). These costs included lost productivity due to crime, illness, and death, as well as added costs in health care and the criminal justice system.

■ STIGMA

Stigma is a negative social value associated with a personal attribute that has consequences in thoughts, emotions, and/or behaviors (e.g., ascribing blame, feeling shame or embarrassment, being shunned and avoided by others) (Link et al. 1997). Many psychiatric and medical conditions carry stigma in our society. Stigma affects the perception and treatment of addiction at multiple decision points, including legislative, judicial, and clinical. Stigma primarily involves the ethical principle of respect for persons, but it becomes a fairness issue when it affects decision making.

The stigma associated with having an addiction is of a particular kind, owing to the fact that addictive behaviors look like, are believed by many to be, and in some (but not all) respects are, voluntary behaviors (Table 8–2). A close parallel in medicine with respect to apparent voluntariness is overeating and obesity. To the extent that a behavior is held to be a voluntary choice made by a free individual, the individual may be held responsible for or blamed for the behavior and its consequences.

TABLE 8–2.	**Sources of stigma in addictions**

- Individuals and society may judge addiction to be fully voluntary; thus, questions about moral accountability arise.
- Use of illicit substances or misuse of legal substances has legal implications and is considered to be immoral by many in society.
- Addictions are perceived to be associated with other stigmatized conditions, such as HIV, hepatitis, homelessness, criminality, and prostitution.
- Within the medical profession, addictions are associated with negative health consequences that carry heavy societal burdens, such as sexually transmitted and infectious diseases, liver failure, heavy emergency service use, and suicidal or self-destructive acts.
- Addictions are associated with negative behaviors or stressors, such as driving under the influence of substances, domestic violence, unemployment, school dropout, and theft.
- Addictions evoke negative cultural and psychological responses, such as fear, disgust, and rejection.

Another major element of the stigma associated with addiction is that substance use itself is often considered morally bad and is often illegal. This element of moral condemnation is also active in the stigma associated with medical disorders such as HIV, where having the disorder implies or suggests behavior (male homosexual behavior and/or intravenous drug use) that some people consider immoral. Persons addicted to illicit drugs are, by definition, criminals. It is a fact that addiction is associated with a number of other behaviors that are considered morally wrong by many or most people (e.g., violence, theft, prostitution, drunk driving, other forms of irresponsibility and negligence). Although many addicted individuals engage in none these behaviors and many nonaddicted persons engage in all of them, there is a tendency for people to make assumptions about the character of addicted individuals on the basis of either accurate or exaggerated knowledge of these associations.

A third major source of stigma is the negative affective responses that people may have to individuals with addictions. These feelings are highly individual and may include reactions such as fear, anger, and avoidance, depending on the individual's psychological makeup. Again, such feelings are aroused by many other medical and psychiatric disorders as well as addiction.

■ PARITY

Parity refers to equitable treatment and equitable access to health care resources according to some consistent criterion. Parity is thus primarily related to the ethical principle of fairness. There is room for debate about the requirements of fairness in health care. There are several approaches that different people might consider fair. For example, health care resource allocation may be based on ability to pay (for insurance or directly for services). In this case, health care is seen as an industry governed by market forces, with minimal government involvement. Alternatively, resource allocation may occur according to need (severity, acuity), or it may derive from the utilitarian principle of maximizing benefit to individuals and to society.

Our present system embodies elements of all three of these models without a single coherent organizing principle. Many public and private health plans provide limited or no coverage for treatment of addictions. Congress is currently debating legislation that would require health plans to provide equal coverage (relative to medical illnesses) for all DSM-IV psychiatric illnesses with the exception of substance use disorders. Such discriminatory policies have been justified by pragmatism: it is argued that full coverage would be prohibitively expensive or politically impossible.

Nevertheless, substance use disorders represent valid, treatable disorders that often have a genetic basis. Health care costs should not be controlled by arbitrarily excluding treatment of particular disorders. It would be just as irrational to exclude treatment of diabetes in order to contain costs.

Returning to the three possible models of fair allocation of health care, whereas market forces may in part determine whether a person has health insurance and his or her overall level of coverage, such forces generally have little to do with the particulars of the coverage or the question of parity. Consistent application of either of the other two models (need-based and utilitarian) would lead to appropriate resource allocation for addiction services. In terms of acuity and severity, addictive disorders cause morbidity and mortality comparable to those of mental illnesses such as depression (Harris and Barraclough 1998). The morbidity caused by substance abuse is immense; an estimated 40 million illnesses and injuries each year are attributable to addiction (McGinnis and Foege 1999). A study conducted in Canada in 1996 found that use of alcohol, tobacco, and illicit drugs accounted for 22.2% years of potential life lost and 9.4% of admissions to hospitals (Single et al. 2000). Finally, in utilitarian terms, addictions are clearly treatable, frequently demonstrating large treatment effects that compare favorably with those of treatment of medical illnesses such as diabetes or hypertension, with benefits to individuals and to society (McLellan et al. 2000). Addiction treatment costs money, but it is not more expensive than treatment of other illnesses, and cost offsets (e.g., from increased productivity, decreased crime, decreased medical costs) are substantial and, according to some studies, considerably greater than the cost of treatment. For example, one study involving 150,000 members of a California health plan found that every $1 spent on substance abuse treatment saved taxpayers $7 in future costs (Gerstein et al. 1997). Given the clear severity of addictive disorders and the relative efficacy of addiction treatment, the only remaining argument against parity for addiction treatment is that addictions are not valid disorders in the sense that major depression and diabetes are. This usually comes down to the argument that substance use is a voluntary behavior and therefore is simply a matter of personal responsibility.

■ PERSONAL RESPONSIBILITY

Although choice certainly plays a role in addictive behavior, important factors beyond personal choice are clearly involved. There is overwhelming evidence that addictive disorders have a biological basis, including genetic inheritance of risk, neurochemical correlates of risk and of active addiction, early recovery, brain reward, and craving states. Many other disorders similarly involve behaviors that seem to be voluntary but that must be dealt with as symptoms of the disorder or as determinants of illness. To continue with the examples used previously, consider diet and medication compliance in diabetes, or suicidal behavior in depression. Categorizing behavior as purely voluntary or involuntary does not correspond to observed reality and distracts from the primary treatment goal of reducing harm.

The issue of personal responsibility is a perplexing one in behavioral health treatment, in that practitioners frequently must grapple with the question of how much to hold a patient accountable for his or her actions and how much to attribute those actions to the patient's illness. One useful way of dealing with this issue is to recognize that responsibility is ultimately an attribution rather than an observable phenomenon. Whether to hold a person responsible is a value judgment based on explicit or implicit values and psychological theories. For clinicians with the primary goals of treating illness, reducing or preventing harm, and/or maximizing wellness, the most appropriate criterion for attributing responsibility is the therapeutic one: attributing responsibility on the basis of therapeutic effect on the patient. Will it be more helpful to the patient to be held responsible for his or her actions, and if so, to what degree? Issues such as limit setting and treatment contracts can be addressed by means of this criterion. Of course the issue of potential harm to others must also be considered and taken into account. Thus, beneficence, fairness, and respect for persons are all involved in the ethical attribution of responsibility.

■ CRIMINAL JUSTICE INVOLVEMENT, TRUTH TELLING, AND CONFIDENTIALITY

Patients with substance use disorders have particularly high rates of criminal justice system involvement. A number of ethical issues arise in the treatment of such patients, which are most effectively dealt with by remembering that the clinician has a primary responsibility to try to help the patient and an additional responsibility to try to prevent harm to others. Beneficence (both toward the patient and toward society at large) and respect for the patient must be balanced in situations in which the patient has already lost some of his or her civil rights.

Patients with criminal justice system involvement may be adjudicated, may have a parole or probation officer (PO) without specific treatment participation requirement, or may be involved in treatment pretrial. In any of these cases, information may be requested from the clinician (e.g., by POs, judges, pretrial supervisors) regarding substance use, participation in treatment, psychiatric status, and the like. Because truthful reporting of information may have negative consequences for the patient, the clinician may experience tension among the conflicting demands of truth telling, confidentiality, and beneficence. One helpful way to think about this dilemma is to recognize that the patient's autonomy and confidentiality are generally compromised primarily by his criminal justice system involvement and only secondarily by his involvement in treatment. In our society, people who have violated the rights of others through criminal behavior may lose some of their civil rights. Truthful-reporting requirements in fact usually have significant positive consequences for the patient. Given that documentation of treatment compliance is often a condition of release, such contact can literally keep the patient out of jail. The patient would be unable to receive and benefit from treatment if the reporting requirement were not met. Such requirements, moreover, serve as a strong, albeit coercive, incentive to participate in treatment. Patients in court-ordered treatment clearly benefit from such treatment.

In the treatment of criminal justice system patients, it is particularly important at the outset of treatment to discuss both with the patient and with any authorities involved the limitations to autonomy and confidentiality that may apply. The patient, even if adjudicated, must provide informed consent to treatment. There is a limitation to this consent, in that treatment may be to some degree coerced and is therefore not fully voluntary. Still, the patient does have the option of refusing treatment and suffering the consequences (e.g., incarceration). The potential risks of treatment (e.g., reporting of noncompliance, resulting in incarceration) should be discussed, and, if the patient is willing, consent for sharing of specific information with the PO or other authority should be obtained. In general, if the form of treatment for the patient is negotiable, the clinician should attempt to limit reporting to the patient's compliance, attainment of general treatment goals, and violent or dangerous behavior. This agreement should be clear to the patient, PO, and clinician. By allowing the clinician honestly to withhold certain information that could be harmful to the patient, such an agreement decreases the potential for conflict between the principles of truth telling and beneficence. In particular, reporting of specific substance use should be avoided, because such a requirement encourages the patient to lie to the clinician if using. The PO or other authority can take responsibility for monitoring substance use by regularly obtaining urine drug screens.

A variety of other situations exist in which truth telling and beneficence can come into conflict in the treatment of patients with addictions. Some of these involve the obligations of compliance with law—for example, reporting an airplane pilot with serious addiction issues or a patient who insists on driving away from the clinic drunk. Other situations have to do with the intersection of therapeutic and justice issues—for example, the temptation to refrain from accurately documenting and assessing a liver transplant candidate who continues to use alcohol or injection drugs.

■ "FIRST, DO NO HARM"

Another issue relating to beneficence is the physician's concern about causing harm by prescribing medication, by causing or enabling addiction, or by causing dangerous interactions with substances of abuse. The idea of providing access to addictive substances challenges physicians' basic sense of the caregiving role, particularly when we prescribe these substances for patients who have substance use disorders. The rationale for such prescribing is evidence-driven and essentially pragmatic: we do it if it helps. For example, for patients with opioid addiction, methadone treatment clearly does much more good than harm. Clinicians frequently avoid using benzodiazepines for anxiety disorders in patients with a history of substance use disorder out of concern that these agents carry a high risk of addiction in such patients. However, this belief is grounded in ideology rather than data: there is little empirical evidence that such patients are at elevated risk of benzodiazepine addiction (Posternak and Mueller 2001). Although a review of pharmacotherapy for patients with addictions is beyond the scope of this chapter, we note that it is generally possible to treat psychiatric disorders in the presence of active substance use disorders. The primary strategy is to reduce morbidity of the psychiatric disorder. Treatment of comorbid psychiatric disorders may improve the outcome of the substance use disorder in some cases and may also serve as a bridge to addiction treatment. Among the addictive disorders, effective pharmacological treatments are currently available only for alcohol, opioid, and nicotine dependence, although medications are frequently used for symptomatic treatment of intoxication and withdrawal from a wider range of substances. Decisions about the use of these medications should be made by applying the same kind of risk–benefit analysis and informed consent process used for any other medication. There is no evidence that any of the approved medications "enable" addiction or compromise recovery.

■ HARM REDUCTION

The concept of harm reduction has engendered considerable controversy among those who believe that abstinence is the only acceptable goal of addiction treatment. The term has been applied to a wide range of interventions and strategies that aim to decrease substance use or the harmful consequences of use rather than focusing on abstinence as the only acceptable goal. From an ethical perspective, the reduction of harm clearly is inherently good unless it secondarily causes other harms. In that case, the secondary harm might be a reduction of the probability of the more highly valued outcome of total abstinence. On the one hand, the concept of harm reduction is an empirical question: there is no evidence that harm-reduction programs such as needle exchange decrease rates of abstinence. On the other hand, it is an ideological question relating to the value of abstinence versus various levels of substance use. One will come to different conclusions if one sees recovery as black and white, abstinent or using, than if one assigns a continuum of values to a continuum of outcomes.

■ PSEUDOADDICTION AND PAIN MANAGEMENT

Management of analgesic addiction in the context of pain syndromes requires heightened sensitivity to ethical considerations, an awareness of the importance of clinician bias, avoidance of stigma, and conscientiousness to the duty of thorough evaluation and careful documentation. A patient seeking drugs because she enjoys them and a patient seeking drugs because she is in pain look and behave much the same. Physicians must be as careful not to induce difficult power struggles related to medication seeking by undertreating pain as they are not to cavalierly dispense addicting substances simply because states license them to do so. In every community, certain doctors are more quick to prescribe, sometimes with no more rationale than the patient's request for a particular drug. Conversely, however, there are also doctors who refuse to prescribe pain medication or who undertreat pain for fear of creating addiction. Adequate treatment of pain syndromes requires spending enough time with the patient to understand the sources of both emotional and physical pain and having the ability to tell the difference. For example, patients with coexisting mood disorders frequently find that they can better tolerate pain when their depression is adequately treated, and vice versa. By the same token, patients often find that when they can give voice to emotional hurts, tolerating physical pain becomes easier. It is irresponsible to treat either pain or addiction as an all-or-none phenomenon (i.e., by prescribing enough medication "no questions asked" to eliminate the pain or by refusing altogether to prescribe addictive medications).

■ EMPIRICAL ETHICS STUDIES

Although many of the ethical considerations in addiction—such as the importance of respect, of fairness, and of minimizing harm—are conceptual, many are issues that could be clarified through empirical data. For example, to what extent can people struggling with addiction provide informed consent at different stages of illness? How does substance dependence affect decisional capacity and voluntarism? Does the effect vary by type of substance? What are the real problems experienced in protecting the confidentiality of people with addictions? How does stigma alter the practices of clinicians who work with individuals with addiction and comorbid disorders? How does stigma affect the attitudes of medical students and residents who might consider career paths in the area of addiction?

Nevertheless, there exist very few empirical studies of ethical issues in addiction treatment. A study that examined informed consent practices among federally funded clinical investigators in the drug and alcohol field (McCrady and Bux 1999) found that two-thirds of the 91 respondents (51% response rate) who completed the survey reported using objective methods to determine participants' ability to provide informed consent. Less than half indicated that they routinely informed study participants of limits to confidentiality in situations of suicidality, homicidality, or child abuse. A substantial minority of the investigators reported experience with these situations in conducting research. Studies in college students have suggested that moral beliefs about substance use influence substance use behavior and that the degree of consistency between moral views and substance use increases with increasing moral maturity within Kohlberg's hierarchy (Abide et al. 2001). A qualitative study has outlined ethical dilemmas arising in work with intravenous drug users (Buchanan et al. 2002). A study of patients entering cocaine treatment found that coercive pressures were pervasive and that "informal psychosocial pressures" were more important than pressures from the legal system in stimulating the request for treatment (Marlowe et al. 1996). Clearly, there is a need for much more empirical work on the ethics of addictions treatment and research.

The field of addiction treatment requires clinicians to deal with a number of complex ethical issues. Although some of these issues are particularly prominent in addiction treatment, most of them are significant in other fields as well. The underlying ethical principles of beneficence, fairness, respect for persons, and truth telling are the same in all areas of medicine.

Case Scenarios

A 42-year-old man with paranoid schizophrenia and heroin dependence, a long history of noncompliance with medications, and initially no interest in addiction treatment was gradually engaged through his case manager's willingness to work with him on an application for disability. The patient eventually was stabilized on antipsychotic medication and entered a methadone program. He has been living independently and clean from illicit drugs for more than a year.

A 22-year-old female has opioid dependence, cocaine and cannabis abuse, and posttraumatic stress disorder (PTSD) resulting from a kidnapping and repeated rape 4 months prior to presentation for treatment. Her PTSD symptoms are severe, and she needs help with case management for her legal problems and unstable housing. However, she misses most of her psychiatric medication and therapy appointments and also takes her methadone irregularly, and she does not seem to be benefiting from treatment. The treatment team repeatedly states its expectation that the patient participate more consistently in treatment but is reluctant to discharge her for noncompliance. After 6 months, she drops out of treatment.

A 43-year-old man with cocaine and alcohol dependence, who is now in parole after serving 9 months on felony assault charges, is court-ordered for treatment. He reports that he has been clean and sober in outpatient treatment for 4 months, but then admits to using cocaine with an old girlfriend twice in a 1-week period. The counselor recommends intensive outpatient treatment, but the PO detects cocaine on a urine drug screen and sends the patient to jail for 1 week. Upon release, the patient undergoes 12 weeks of intensive outpatient treatment and remains clean and compliant with treatment for the remainder of 18 months' probation.

Case Scenarios *(continued)*

A 37-year-old man has a 20-year history of alcohol dependence and a 2-year history of cognitive impairment due to a head injury sustained in an assault. Now he is impulsive, emotionally labile, lacking in judgment and planning ability, and chronically suicidal, and he continues to drink alcohol at every opportunity. After several unsuccessful attempts by physicians to have him committed to long-term treatment, a legal guardian is named. However, the patient wanders away from group homes and nursing homes, and he is eventually found beaten to death on the street.

A 39-year-old woman with alcohol dependence and severe panic disorder, who has been sober for 4 years but continues to use marijuana regularly, has been maintained on relatively high doses of clonazepam for panic disorder. After her daughter runs away from home, the patient relapses on alcohol and is hospitalized for detoxification. She is started on disulfiram (Antabuse), and with some trepidation her psychiatrist restarts the clonazepam to treat her emergent panic attacks. The patient remains sober 9 months later but continues so smoke marijuana.

■ REFERENCES

Abide MM, Richards HC, Ramsay SG: Moral reasoning and consistency of belief and behavior: decisions about substance abuse. J Drug Educ 31:367–384, 2001

American Psychiatric Association: Diagnostic and Statistical Manual of Mental Disorders, 4th Edition, Text Revision. Washington, DC, American Psychiatric Association, 2000

Buchanan D, Khoshnood K, Stopka T, et al: Ethical dilemmas created by the criminalization of status behaviors: case examples from ethnographic field research with injection drug users. Health Educ Behav 29:30–42, 2002

Gerstein DR, Johnson RA, Larison CL: Alcohol and Drug Treatment Outcomes for Patients and Welfare Recipients: Outcomes, Benefits, and Costs. Washington, DC, U.S. Department of Health and Human Services, Office of the Secretary for Planning and Evaluation, 1997

Harris EC, Barraclough B: Excess mortality of mental disorder. Br J Psychiatry 173:11–53, 1998

Kessler RC, McGonagle KA, Zhao S, et al: Lifetime and 12-month prevalence of DSM-III-R psychiatric disorders in the United States. Results from the National Comorbidity Survey. Arch Gen Psychiatry 51:8–19, 1994

Link BG, Struening EL, Rahav M, et al: On stigma and its consequences: evidence from a longitudinal study of men with dual diagnoses of mental illness and substance abuse. J Health Soc Behav 38:177–190, 1997

Marlowe DB, Kirby KC, Bonieskie M, et al: Assessment of coercive and noncoercive pressures to enter drug abuse treatment. Drug Alcohol Depend 42:77–84, 1996

McCrady BS, Bux DA Jr: Ethical issues in informed consent with substance abusers. J Consult Clin Psychol 67:186–193, 1999

McGinnis JM, Foege WH: Mortality and morbidity attributable to use of addictive substances in the United States. Proc Assoc Am Physicians 111: 109–118, 1999

McLellan AT, Lewis DC, O'Brien CP, et al: Drug dependence, a chronic medical illness: implications for treatment, insurance, and outcomes evaluation. JAMA 284:1689–1695, 2000

National Household Survey on Drug Abuse. Washington, DC, Substance Abuse and Mental Health Services Administration, 1999

Posternak MA, Mueller TI: Assessing the risks and benefits of benzodiazepines for anxiety disorders in patients with a history of substance abuse or dependence. Am J Addict 10:48–68, 2001

Regier DA, Narrow WE, Rae DS, et al: The de facto US mental and addictive disorders service system. Epidemiologic Catchment Area prospective 1-year prevalence rates of disorders and services. Arch Gen Psychiatry 50:85–94, 1993

Rice DP, Kelman S, Miller LS: Estimates of economic costs of alcohol and drug abuse and mental illness, 1985 and 1988. Public Health Rep 106: 280–292, 1991

Single E, Rehm J, Robson L, et al: The relative risks and etiologic fractions of different causes of death and disease attributable to alcohol, tobacco and illicit drug use in Canada. CMAJ 162:1669–1675, 2000

9

CARING FOR
"DIFFICULT" PATIENTS

There are patients, and there are patients. The difficult ones can be "demanding," "noncompliant," "whiny," "entitled," or "manipulative." They can be too different from or too similar to the clinician, too seductive, too unclean, too smart, too fat, too thin, or too anxiety-provoking (McCarty and Roberts 1996). These patients require special attention because their care is very complex and because it invites significant ethical pitfalls. Recognizing what makes some patients "difficult," understanding that "being difficult" is a clinical sign that warrants diagnostic interpretation, identifying the special ethical problems arising in the care of the difficult patient, and responding therapeutically are the key elements of ethically sound care for these challenging patients.

■ RECOGNIZING "DIFFICULT" PATIENTS

It is often obvious who is, or is going to become, difficult. The patient who is perceived as "drug seeking," the patient who is notorious for not taking his medications, the patient who engages in frequent self-mutilating behavior, the patient who seems to complain incessantly, the patient who threatens violence toward clinic staff, the patient who demands discharge from the hospital, the patient who is "just a personality disorder," the patient who seems never to get better—these are the tough cases.

Sometimes the difficult patients can be more subtle in their presentation, however. The patient with a professional background who is utterly bright and engaging may end up being very difficult because he relates to the clinician as a friend from whom he asks for "favors" of prescriptions and laboratory tests. Similarly, the care of a patient who is also a clinician may become especially complex, for several reasons. For example, the patient may feel ashamed to reveal his health issues to a professional colleague. On the other hand, the caregiver may assume that the clinician/patient needs less support and reassurance than other patients. The caregiver may also fail to explore the possibility of self-diagnosis and self-prescribing by the clinician/patient. Other subtly difficult patients include individuals who omit or obscure important details when providing their histories and those who, along with their multiple medical and psychiatric symptoms, have multiple caregivers and multiple ongoing treatments.

Recognizing the difficult patient, then, involves identifying those individuals who are unusual in one of two ways. First, these patients may be difficult because of the special intensity of feelings (i.e., countertransference) they evoke by the clinical care team. For example, the patient whom one is especially tempted to "rescue," to identify with, or to feel awed by is likely to be difficult. The victimized child, the physician/patient, the parish priest or local television news anchor, and people who look like the clinician's Uncle Joe, Cousin Mary, or fifth grade teacher Mrs. Panturo may all fit into this category. Worse yet are patients who actually *are* the clinician's Uncle Joe, Cousin Mary, or fifth grade teacher Mrs. Panturo—a phenomenon that is not unusual in some small towns or small health care systems. The patient who is also a litigation attorney may be a particularly intimidating—and therefore challenging—patient for any caregiver. The patient who has extraordinarily severe symptoms may be perceived as a difficult patient if he evokes feelings of distress or inadequacy in the clinician.

Other patients who present special problems are those whose experiences and illness processes are so tragic that they engender very powerful feelings of empathy and pain in their caregivers. These are the patients that clinicians carry with them, that make clinicians lose sleep, that clinicians always remember. The young mother dying of cancer, the military colonel who gradually succumbs to Alzheimer's disease, the newly quadriplegic motorcycle accident victim, the survivor of wartime torture and trauma, the child who has been raped, and the college student who attempts suicide during his first psychotic break—these are the patients whom clinicians and clinical trainees may find very overwhelming and for whom they may find it extraordinarily difficult to provide effective care.

Patients who trigger unusually strong negative feelings ("gut reactions") from members of the staff are also likely to present special challenges. These reactions may be due to the particular problematic feelings and conduct (e.g., anger, emotional lability, inconsistency, indifference, repeated suicide threats, self-mutilating or self-defeating behaviors) and psychological defenses (e.g., denial, projection, reaction formation) of the patients. They may also be related to uncomfortable or stigmatizing elements of a patient's personal life history, such as the gang member who has served time in prison, the father whose careless driving resulted in the death of his child in an accident, or the pregnant woman who uses methadone. An unusual physical appearance—such as obesity, cachexia, exceptionally poor hygiene, congenital abnormalities, or regions of infection—may also trigger such feelings in caregivers. In some instances, the clinical care team will react to a given patient with disinterest and detachment. Although less overt than other "strong" negative reactions, such detachment likewise is an indicator of a problematic patient. The clinician who is well attuned to his or her own emotional responses, and those of the patient care team, will thus be well prepared to identify these difficult patients.

Beyond these affective factors that make a given patient unusual, a second cue in recognizing difficult patients is their atypical pattern of clinical service use. Patients who appear to seek prescription medications from many sources, to be overly insistent about clinic appointments and specialty referrals, or to obtain care repeatedly through emergency or urgent care facilities will come to be experienced as difficult patients by their care providers. Patients who appear to emphasize physical symptoms in mental health care settings and mental health symptoms in physical health care settings are particularly apt to stymie their caregivers. These patients often suffer from several comorbid physical and mental illness processes, giving rise to this kind of service utilization pattern. In contrast, the "underutilizers" of clinical services, such as patients who present late in the course of illness for treatment, demand discharge from the hospital against medical advice (AMA), do not take their medications, miss their scheduled appointments, or do not pursue necessary preventive care (e.g., parents who do not arrange for their children to receive appropriate vaccinations) will also pose special challenges and arouse strong emotions in caregivers. Such patients have been described as "help rejecters" (Robbins et al. 1988). Clinical syndromes may be the direct "cause" of these impaired care-seeking behaviors, as in the case of the social phobic patient or the negative-symptom-dominant schizophrenia patient with numerous "no shows" for clinic appointments. Similarly, the cardiac patient with an unrecognized alcohol problem may place his caregivers in clinical and ethical binds by insisting on leaving the hospital prematurely as he finds his withdrawal symptoms harder to tolerate.

■ PREVALENCE AND ATTRIBUTES OF "DIFFICULT" PATIENTS IN MEDICAL AND PSYCHIATRIC SETTINGS

Because difficult patients take so many different forms, their relative numbers are difficult to estimate accurately. In medical settings, roughly one-sixth of patient encounters are perceived by clinicians as involving "difficult patients" (Jackson and Kroenke 1999). In one study of 500 patients, 15% were identified by their primary care providers as "difficult," and these patients were more likely to have mental disorders, more than 5 somatic symptoms, more severe symptoms, poorer functional status, lesser satisfaction with care, and higher use of health services (Jackson and Kroenke 1999). In this study, physicians with more negative psychosocial attitudes as measured on the Physician's Belief Scale were significantly more likely to experience patient encounters as difficult. In another study of 293 patients presenting for care in medical and surgical clinics, 22% were identified by consultants as leading to "difficult encounters," primarily due to medically unexplained symptoms, coexisting social problems, and severe, untreatable illness (Sharpe et al. 1994). Encounter difficulty was associated with greater patient distress, less patient satisfaction, and heightened use of services.

A third study of 113 patients similarly found that difficult patients were characterized by psychosomatic symptoms, at least mild personality disorder, addiction, and major psychopathology (e.g., affective or anxiety disorders) but that demographic characteristics, provider characteristics, and most diagnoses were not correlated with a higher score on the Difficult Doctor–Patient Relationship Questionnaire (Hahn et al. 1994). In a study of 43 patients (21 identified as "difficult" and 22 controls), structured diagnostic evaluation revealed that a greater number of the difficult patients (7 of 21 vs. 1 of 22) had personality disorders. Five of the difficult patients with personality disorders met criteria for "dependent" personality, and none had had this psychopathology diagnosed previously (Schafer and Nowlis 1998). These findings echo those of a more recent study in which borderline personality disorder was found to be present in patients at an urban primary care clinic at four times the prevalence found in community populations (Gross et al. 2002). Half of these patients had received no mental health treatment, and 43% had not been accurately diagnosed in their primary care clinic. Other factors that may contribute to difficult patient encounters, such as perceived deception by patients, have been studied only minimally. However, one interesting study that assessed patient encounters of 44 family practice residents and attending physicians revealed that clinicians commonly doubted the truthfulness of their patients' disclosures (19.5% and 8.7%, respectively) (Woolley and Clements 1997).

Analogous data have not been collected systematically in mental health care settings. Treatment resistance and nonadherence, very heavy utilization of mental health services, severe psychopathology due to personality disorders or psychotic disorders, and comorbid disease have been suggested as causes of difficult encounters in psychiatric settings (Hahn et al. 1996). The prevalence of difficult patient encounters is likely to be significantly higher in mental health care than in traditional medical settings, because of the specific nature of psychiatric illness and its care. Our patients have illnesses that affect behaviors, personal attitudes, mood symptoms, insight and motivation, and decision making. They have complex psychosocial issues, and the sicker patients often are poor and have limited abilities and/or opportunities to improve their socioeconomic circumstances. Patients with personality disorders who ultimately are referred for mental health treatment tend to be very seriously disturbed, and their care poses immense challenges. Patients with a constellation of medical and mental health symptoms who are referred for psychiatric consultation also tend to be very distressed, to pose diagnostic enigmas, or to have especially overwhelming psychosocial issues. For these reasons, mental health practitioners may feel that every patient encounter will potentially become a difficult one.

■ UNDERSTANDING "DIFFICULT" AS A CLINICAL SIGN

The clinician's first duty in the care of the difficult patient is to understand that the aspects of the patient's presentation that make him or her "difficult" are, in essence, clinical signs—that is, observable manifestations of the patient's underlying health and of factors affecting his or her health status. In other words, there is a differential diagnosis that accompanies "being difficult." The patient who is threatening in his behavior toward clinic staff may in fact be experiencing irritability, fear, and psychotic symptoms early in the course of a manic episode. The patient could also be head-injured, delirious, or intoxicated. The frustratingly "noncompliant" patient with unremitting symptoms may hold different religious beliefs about acceptable healing practices, may have experienced unpleasant side effects of pills, may not have insight about the need for treatment, or, alternatively, may not have the resources to purchase prescription medications or to obtain transportation for clinic appointments. Moreover, because traumatized individuals often tend to relive their past experiences in the context of their current lives, the patient who behaves seductively in the therapeutic relationship may have been sexually exploited in the past. Rather than expressing authentic romantic feelings for the clinician, this patient is manifesting his or her core psychological issues for the clinician, who has the duty to understand this clinical phenomenon. Such "difficult" behaviors should be understood in a dispassionate, nonjudgmental manner. They are observable clinical "signs."

Clarifying the reasons why patients appear to be undermining their own health and health care is therefore an important responsibility of the clinician. Behavioral cues of patients should be explored and interpreted clinically, not superficially or too concretely. Just as the seductive patient should not be taken at face value, the angry patient also should not be viewed as intentionally "acting out" in order to "create trouble." In sum, all elements of the patient's presentation are important clinical data, and clinicians must remain within their professional roles and uphold their professional duties when dealing with the challenges of the difficult patient.

■ IDENTIFYING ETHICAL PITFALLS IN THE CARE OF DIFFICULT PATIENTS

Difficult patients are at risk of receiving care that deviates from usual ethics standards in several respects. First, therapeutic abandonment of patients is much more likely when they are unlikable, frustrating, apparently noncompliant, extraordinarily tragic, or otherwise atypical. Efforts made to preserve the therapeutic alliance and to obtain appropriate informed refusal of treatment with a patient who is "medication seeking" or "demanding AMA discharge" may be minimal in many circumstances, for instance. The caregiver may pay less attention to carefully diagnosing the multiple clinical problems of the patient whose interpersonal manner and use of health services are seen as "inappropriate." Important medical issues that merit exploration may be dismissed as "psychiatric," as, for example, in the situation of a medical student with undiagnosed Crohn's disease whose symptoms are attributed to exam-related stress and poor coping skills. Gradual, quiet disengagement from the persistently suffering patient, although not legally problematic, is another subtle form of therapeutic abandonment that may occur.

Second, professional boundaries may erode in the care of difficult patients, resulting in ethically compromised care. When patients are difficult because they resemble their caregivers in terms of having similar backgrounds, professions, or interests, the clinician and patient may begin relating to one another in a manner more congruent with a friendship than a professional relationship—for example, the clinician may disclose aspects of his or her personal life, accept financial advice, or make social plans in the course of talking with the patient. Personal–professional boundaries are crossed in such situations, and the ethical foundation of the relationship—trust and absolute dedication to the well-being of the patient—may be seriously jeopardized. Informed consent processes may suffer, because these clinicians may provide insufficient information about clinical care alternatives or may suggest only those treatment options that they personally would consider. Caregivers who overly identify with their patients may also be tempted to document clinical issues inaccurately or to not comply with legal mandatory-reporting duties when stigmatizing issues arise in such cases. Splits within treatment teams may occur as some clinicians become closer to difficult patients for whom they have warmer personal feelings and other members of the team do not. Clinicians may act unprofessionally in subtle ways by providing undocumented prescriptions or samples of medications. They may also act unprofessionally in more overt ways by becoming intimately involved with patients who give sexualized behavioral cues or who are otherwise vulnerable to the approaches of a "powerful" person.

Third, confidentiality breaches may occur when caregivers discuss the difficult patient's case in relatively public settings, a behavior fueled by strongly held and hard-to-contain feelings. The temptation to discuss the case is especially acute when the patient is an aggravating individual about whom the clinical team has passionate complaints, but it is also an issue when, for example, the patient is a celebrity or a celebrity's child who suffers from a serious mental illness and/or substance problems. It is often difficult for clinicians to manage their natural curiosity, even voyeurism, and their desire to discuss the patient with colleagues and friends in such cases.

The challenges in caring for difficult patients therefore affect every ethically important aspect of clinical practice. Maintaining attentiveness to the clinical signs and symptoms of the patient, building and sustaining the therapeutic alliance, respecting the autonomy of the patient through sound informed consent and refusal-of-treatment processes, upholding the law, and maintaining appropriate confidentiality safeguards may all be adversely affected.

■ RESPONDING THERAPEUTICALLY

Ensuring that difficult patients receive clinically and ethically sound care is no small task (Table 9–1). The most critical step in responding therapeutically is to recognize the discomfort and problems that difficult patients generate as a clinical sign (Figure 9–1). Monitoring one's own reactions and responding with professionalism and thoroughness to the symptoms and behavioral presentations of these special patients are the keys to providing good care in potentially taxing clinical situations. Responding therapeutically may entail building a sense of empathy for the unlikable or otherwise off-putting patient; it may entail assuming a more professional, more objective stance with the especially charming or intriguing patient.

Several core elements of treatment for the difficult patient have been proposed by experienced clinicians (Drossman 1978; McCarty and Roberts 1996). These include maintaining a nonjudgmental interest in the patient's reports; keeping personal and professional roles "straight"; reflecting on one's own attitudes and biases; taking a complete history and accepting (not arguing with or discounting) the patient's symptoms; performing or referring the patient for a thorough physical examination; avoiding patronizing or inappropriate reassurance ("it's just stress"); refraining from intervening with medications or aggressive treatments prematurely; setting up regular visits and being interpersonally "predictable" and consistent; remaining alert for new developments; clearly presenting therapeutic

TABLE 9–1.   **Steps in managing difficult patients**

Step 1: Understand yourself

Be aware of your own biases and responses.

Understand why certain types of patients upset you.

Realize you're not a "bad" doctor if you have negative feelings about some patients.

Recognize that everyone has trouble managing some patients.

Step 2: Understand your patient

Every difficult behavior is a form of communication.

Every difficult patient is trying to express real fears and needs.

Step 3: Think, don't react

Remember your duty to help and not harm.

Focus on medical and psychiatric issues you can treat.

Strive to be empathic, consistent, and stable.

Step 4: Form an alliance

Find something you can agree upon.

Educate the patient about your limits and responsibilities.

Reinforce positive behavior, don't reward negative behavior.

Step 5: Treat whatever is treatable

Screen for medical conditions.

Screen for Axis I and Axis II disorders.

Use therapy and medication to treat problems.

Step 6: Avoid the traps

Of wanting to save the patient and be idealized.

Of wanting to reject the patient and not be hurt.

Of wanting to punish the patient.

Of doing anything to help the patient so he won't hurt himself.

Step 7: Get help

Seek consultation.

Foster team consensus.

Encourage patient to participate in support groups.

Step 8: Handle your emotions

Find constructive ways of venting frustration.

Prepare yourself for seeing difficult patients.

See managing difficult patients as a clinical skill to master.

Acknowledgment.   Cynthia M. A. Geppert, M.D., Ph.D., provided assistance in preparing this table.

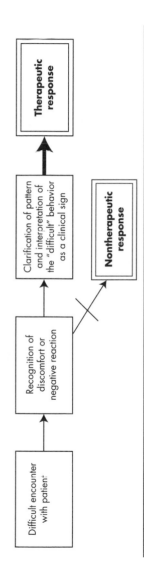

FIGURE 9–1. **Responding therapeutically to the "difficult" patient.**
Source. Adapted from McCarty T, Roberts LW: "The Difficult Patient," in *Medicine: A Primary Care Approach.* Edited by Rubin RH, Voss C, Derksen DJ, et al. Philadelphia, PA, WB Saunders, 1996, p. 397. Used with permission.

options to the patient; preparing for a protracted course of treatment; communicating all findings and treatment plans to the clinical care team before, during, and after their discovery or implementation; and educating oneself about the biopsychosocial aspects of the patient's disease process.

It is also important to accept one's own limitations in dealing with the countertransference and ethical issues presented by difficult patients and to seek out appropriate professional venues for clarifying these issues. For example, thoughtful discussions with members of the clinical care team about strategies for responding to the frustrations encountered in a particular patient's care may be highly valuable. Comparing and double-checking one's own perceptions with those of trusted team members will be a helpful step in this process. Seeking out additional clinical, ethical, and legal expertise from knowledgeable colleagues and supervisors is especially important. Use of humor when discussing highly problematic patients with clinical team members is controversial from an ethical perspective. Although perhaps not optimal, humor is often inevitable in caring for difficult patients and can be put to constructive use in illuminating the more troublesome features of the patient's case and highlighting the powerlessness or frustration felt by members of the clinical team. So long as there are ample manifestations of respect toward the patient and faithfulness to the ethical principles of beneficence and nonmaleficence in the patient's care—*and* a thoughtful discussion of the treatment issues—the team leader may interpret the humor in a manner that contributes positively to the "multiproblem" patient's care.

One final consideration in this challenging process is to examine the lessons learned in the course of caring for difficult patients— the unexpected diagnosis of the patient, the unexpected strengths of a team member, the unexpected impact of a miscommunication, the unexpected community resource, the unexpected resilience of the caregiver. Paying attention to these valuable lessons will help address the natural exhaustion felt by many clinicians, and it will also help expand their repertoire of skills and abilities for their next patient encounter, which may or may not pose special difficulties.

Case Scenarios

A young man with self-mutilating behavior presents to the psychiatric emergency room, having chewed and swallowed glass after being stopped by police for driving while intoxicated.

A young woman with a history of sexual trauma and abnormal menstrual bleeding asks her primary care physician to set up a gynecological examination. Although she has missed her last two appointments, the physician arranges for an appointment for later in the week. She arrives late, says "I'm pregnant," appears distraught, and tells the nurse that she "just took a lot of pills." She is taken to the emergency room.

A senior medical student approaches his supervisor, an attending physician, for antidepressant and sleeping medications. He states that he is under tremendous stress but does not wish to seek formal care because he "can't afford to get a mental health record" if he wants to "get into a residency program."

An elderly man who ordinarily lives in a motel for transients in a poor neighborhood presents to the psychiatric emergency room on a cold winter night, with all of his possessions in a large plastic bag. He demands admission to the hospital, stating that he will kill himself if he is sent to a shelter. The staff note that the patient's pattern is to come to the ER toward the end of the month, when he has run out of money and is unable to stay at his motel.

A recently retired man with mild hypertension, arthritis, and a family history of cancer (both of his parents died of cancer) seems to fill every appointment with a recitation of complaints and worries. Each time the physician tries a different treatment, the patient returns, complaining of its lack of efficacy. The patient frequently discontinues his medications prematurely because of "side effects." He makes frequent calls to the doctor's office and is "known" for his pattern of frequent visits to the urgent care and walk-in clinics.

A veteran with comorbid mental and addictive illnesses is admitted to a psychiatric inpatient unit. Four days into his hospitalization, he is allowed to go on a walk with his brother and sister-in-law on the grounds of the VA facility. He returns 10 minutes late, walking unsteadily and speaking rapidly and in an animated fashion.

■ REFERENCES

Drossman DA: The problem patient: evaluation and care of medical patients with psychosocial disturbances. Ann Intern Med 88:366–372, 1978

Gross R, Olfson M, Gameroff M, et al: Borderline personality disorder in primary care. Arch Intern Med 162:53–60, 2002

Hahn SR, Kroenke K, Spitzer RL, et al: The difficult patient: prevalence, psychopathology, and functional impairment. J Gen Intern Med 11:1–8, 1996

Hahn SR, Thompson KS, Wills TA, et al: The difficult doctor-patient relationship: somatization, personality and psychopathology. J Clin Epidemiol 47:647–657, 1994

Jackson JL, Kroenke K: Difficult patient encounters in the ambulatory clinic: clinical predictors and outcomes. Arch Intern Med 159:1069–1075, 1999

McCarty T, Roberts LW: The difficult patient, in Medicine: A Primary Care Approach. Edited by Rubin RH, Voss C, Derksen DJ, et al. Philadelphia, PA, WB Saunders, 1996, pp 395–399

Robbins JM, Beck PR, Mueller DP, et al: Therapists' perceptions of difficult psychiatric patients. J Nerv Ment Dis 176:490–497, 1988

Schafer S, Nowlis DP: Personality disorders among difficult patients. Arch Fam Med 7:126–129, 1998

Sharpe M, Mayou R, Seagroatt V, et al: Why do doctors find some patients difficult to help? Q J Med 87:187–193, 1994

Woolley D, Clements T: Family medicine residents' and community physicians' concerns about patient truthfulness. Acad Med 72:155–157, 1997

10

CARING FOR PEOPLE IN SMALL COMMUNITIES

Special ethical problems arise in small communities, which can range from family villages in the Alaskan bush, college campuses in Iowa, communities in rural Appalachia, and ethnic enclaves in New York City. *Patients* in these communities are often isolated, have limited access to health care services, hold distinct cultural beliefs related to health and illness, and seek care from clinicians who are also neighbors, friends, family, or professional colleagues. *Clinicians* in these communities struggle with problems inherent to the context—helping to overcome geographic, resource, and/or attitudinal barriers to care; choosing which patients receive which health services; deciding how much to say or not to say in social situations; providing care for one's own sibling or child in an emergency situation; functioning without multidisciplinary specialist support; and coping with their own exhaustion and stresses. Ethical dilemmas of small communities have been poorly recognized and are heightened when stigmatizing disorders (e.g., substance dependence, mental illness) are involved. Furthermore, these dilemmas are not easily remedied by ethics guidelines that derive from larger, richer, and more flexible contexts. Nevertheless, rural clinicians comment on the positive aspects of their work and the important roles they play in caring for patients and families and in serving their communities. Insight into the distinct ethical attributes of small communities and several clinical ethics problem-solving strategies may assist clinicians and trainees working in these special circumstances.

■ ETHICAL DILEMMAS OF SMALL COMMUNITIES

Small-community ethics dilemmas primarily relate to five issues (Table 10–1): 1) overlapping relationships, conflicting roles and altered therapeutic boundaries; 2) confidentiality; 3) cultural dimensions of care; 4) limited access to clinical care, mental health, and ethics resources; and 5) special stresses of small-community clinicians.

Overlapping Relationships, Conflicting Roles, and Altered Therapeutic Boundaries

Overlapping relationships are the rule rather than the exception in small towns: the doctor and the patient grew up on neighboring farms; the clinic nurse attended high school with the patient's daughter; the office manager and the patient are members of the same church; and the patients all talk to one another in the coffee shop while waiting for their appointments. In another "small town," a medical school or college campus, the student may need to seek care from a faculty supervisor or through a "gatekeeping" undergraduate advisor—that is, someone who plays an important educational role in the student's life and may greatly influence his or her future professional opportunities. Especially in more remote, more tightly knit, or more restricted communities, health providers routinely interact with patients in nonmedical, "overlapping" roles.

In one poignant example, a patient drove several hours to a university hospital emergency room for help with his substance abuse problem. He said that he could not seek care "at home" because his sister worked at the mental health clinic. The distance this man was required to travel to obtain care ultimately became burdensome to him and was identified as a reason for the patient's noncompliance with subsequent treatment. The overlapping role with a clinical staff member in this case led to a series of significant barriers for necessary care.

Overlapping relationships are ethically complex because they bring differing roles, duties, and motivations to clinician–patient in-

TABLE 10–1. Small-community ethical problems and solutions

Issue	Problem areas	Solutions
Overlapping relationships: complex and differing roles, duties and motivations brought to clinician–patient relationship	Personal and professional roles routinely overlap in community life	Educate office staff and colleagues about problems with personal/professional relationships in small communities
	Clinicians may be caught in "binds" between serving needs of patient and community	Establish backup arrangements so that team members may be excused from sensitive situations
	Clinicians may have difficulty maintaining therapeutic boundaries	Build a reciprocal referral network in neighboring communities
		Discuss overlapping relationships with patients to minimize impact on care, and separate conflicting roles where possible
Confidentiality: respect for patient privacy	Patients may be uncomfortable seeking treatment for stigmatizing conditions as a result of overlapping relationships	Implement "confidentiality routines" (e.g., keep charts and computers hidden, discuss patient care only behind closed doors, use shadow charts and encoding)
	Office breaches of confidentiality cause harm to patient, such as loss of respect or employment	Follow up leaks of information to reinforce policy of protecting patient privacy
	Patients may not seek care or may leave care prematurely, and the duty to continually "keep secrets" may cause physicians to feel isolated	Provide medical and mental health services through a single clinic to avoid stigma

TABLE 10–1.   Small-community ethical problems and solutions *(continued)*

Issue	Problem areas	Solutions
Cultural issues: values and beliefs affecting recognition of illness, pursuit of care, perception of consent, medical preferences, and views of clinicians and treatment	Mental illnesses may not be culturally sanctioned or may be defined alternatively, and degree of "truth telling" and decision making may differ among cultural groups Ethical mistakes may arise through ignorance or disregard of cultural values An overemphasis on cultural values may lead to ethical mistakes and the erosion of professional values	Enlist the help of community leaders to design culturally effective approaches Be aware of influence of personal cultural beliefs for the clinical role without losing own cultural identity Address clinical mistakes in a culturally congruent manner Communicate decisions—especially when they are at odds with community standards and when the values underlying them are a manifestation of medical necessity and professional integrity

TABLE 10–1. Small-community ethical problems and solutions *(continued)*

Issue	Problem areas	Solutions
Limited access to clinical care: resource limitations in continuity of care, effectiveness of service, and ability and willingness of patients to use services	Rural areas may lack emergency, urgent-care, or special-care facilities or clinicians Nonphysician providers have increased responsibility without additional training Few hospital-based supports—such as ethics committees and consultants and multidisciplinary teams—are available Distance, ethnic and language differences, time of year, and physician openness to alternative treatments all affect actual use of services	Develop collegial relationships for support and guidance Use the Internet and video conferencing to build a consultation network Advocate for and educate others about rural health needs
Small-community clinician stress: unique stresses as a result of overlapping roles, long hours, little support, and isolation	Clinicians who follow their own ethical guidelines may risk ethical and/or legal problems Because specialists often are not available, physicians may practice outside of their expertise Clinician and resource shortages may lead to burnout and cynicism Overlapping roles and distance may result in personal and professional isolation	Identify and minimize career-related stresses and role conflicts Balance practice patterns and caseloads Advocate for and educate others about rural health needs Develop adequate backup coverage to allow vacations Attend to self-care, including physical, emotional, and social health

teractions. Instead of focusing exclusively on the well-being of the patient, for instance, small-community clinicians may feel caught between serving the needs of the individual patient and responding to the needs of their shared community (Simon and Williams 1999). This is apparent in the example of a physician, living adjacent to an Indian rural reservation, who discovered that his patient, a very powerful tribal council member, had sexually abused a number of children nearby. The physician complied with the mandatory reporting law in that state, even though he knew that the tribal council, his employer, and his neighbors and friends in the broader community would be divided about the decision. This is also apparent in the example of the medical school clerkship director who works in the student health clinic and determines that a student-patient has a serious substance dependence problem. Intervening therapeutically, fulfilling mandatory reporting requirements for the state and for the institution, and evaluating the student academically in a fair manner, taken together, are very challenging. In both of these situations, the clinician may make a number of ethical errors of omission (e.g., overlooking the problems identified or failing to report them in compliance with the law) or commission (e.g., using or talking about sensitive personal information derived from the patient encounter in other contexts).

Overlapping relationships also generate ethical problems because of conflicting roles and their adverse effects on treatment boundaries (Perkins et al. 1998). As described in Chapter 3, treatment boundaries are defined as the rules and conduct that establish the professional relationship as distinct from other relationships and as fundamentally respectful and protective of patients (Simon 1992). In some small villages, clinicians must seek goods and services from patients—bartering or bickering over "fair" prices is part of the community culture. Typically, the nature of the relationship between the buyer and the seller influences the terms and process of negotiation. In such circumstances, it is difficult to address the inequalities of the clinician–patient relationship squarely and in a manner that is not exploitative. In another kind of situation, an Alaskan psychiatrist was asked to perform forensic evaluations of his own patients for the state court system because no other doctoral-level mental health professional was available in the region. He felt conflicted about acting as a "dual agent" in this way, because his opinions offered in the service of the court would directly affect the sentencing process. Because of such pressures associated with overlapping roles in small communities, physicians may ultimately—if unknowingly—serve interests and concerns other than those of their patients. In addition, because guidelines followed by centralized licensing boards and by nationally based professional organizations may not reflect attunement to the small-community context, clinicians in small communities may be judged by incorrect standards when claims of ethical misconduct arise.

Confidentiality

Respect for patient privacy is a crucial element of trust in the clinical relationship (see Chapter 7) but, as one rural inhabitant remarked, "We may not have a lot of people—but we sure do have a lot of talk!" Another person who grew up in a small town has commented, "Everybody watches who goes into the clinic on Wednesdays when the mental health counselor visits…heaven forbid that you get a sore throat on Tuesday night!" Particularly when stigmatizing health issues emerge, such as those associated with mental illness, sexuality, relationship stresses, or substance use, small-community residents may become acutely uncomfortable with the prospect of disclosing intimate information to their clinicians. Even when patients overcome this barrier, they may reasonably fear that office staff will learn of their personal health concerns. This is true for rural patients in the doctor's office and college professors at the university health clinic alike. Moreover, it may be a realistic worry, as losses—ranging from respect to employment—may result from confidentiality breaches in the context of a small, closed community. Because of these concerns, patients may not seek necessary care or they may later be lost from the therapeutic alliance. This may be the case even for patients with very serious disorders. This poorly recognized barrier to care was shown in a survey study of

160 multidisciplinary clinicians in Alaska and New Mexico, in which clinicians in smaller communities (population less than 2,500) expressed greater agreement with the statement that confidentiality concerns interfere with patients' willingness to talk openly about sensitive issues (Roberts et al. 2003).

Cultural Dimensions of Care

Cultural issues influence health care in small-community contexts. Cultural values and beliefs affect recognition of illness, pursuit of care, perceptions of informed consent, expression of medical preferences, and attitudes toward caregivers and toward health care interventions. Certain forms of mental illness are not recognized or even given a name in some cultures. Alternative explanations or attributions are proffered instead, such as that the depressed person lacks "moral fiber" (as perceived in some agricultural communities) or that the psychotic person has "witch sickness" because of a spiritual imbalance or problem within the larger community (Zuni people) or because of having failed to undergo ritual cleansing after having come into contact with a corpse (Navajo people). Similarly, how clinical information and guidance is disclosed varies among rural populations. For instance, definitions of physical and psychological health were explored in 62 men and women from 13 rural counties in Montana. Health in this group of individuals was defined as "the ability to work or to be productive in one's role. Ranchers and farmers stated that pain would be tolerated for extended periods so long as it did not interfere [with work].... Mental health problems were rarely mentioned" (Braden and Beauregard 1994). Indeed, individuals from different cultural backgrounds differ in their views of pain, disease concepts and etiological explanations for sicknesses, patterns of use of folk healers and alternative medicines, tolerance of illness, stoicism, and acceptance of technological interventions.

The ethical principles of respect for persons and justice necessitate that care provided in small communities reflect attunement to the cultural beliefs and expectations of both the patient and the community. Cultural ethical mistakes may arise when clinicians manifest unawareness of or disregard for indigenous values and behaviors by, for example, interfering with a healing ceremony, failing to work with the natural supports within families and communities, inappropriately interpreting interpersonal cues on the mental status examination, or disregarding the choices and personal beliefs of a patient. A second kind of ethical mistake may occur when clinicians overemphasize indigenous values to the point of diminishing the clinician's own profession's values and ethics—values and ethics that admittedly have derived from the larger culture but that are the basic guideposts for decision making in most clinical situations. This emphasis, which some authors have referred to as "romanticization" of different cultures, may lead to underdiagnosis and poor treatment of patients. It also may give rise to inadvertent "collusion" with the maladaptive behaviors and coping problems of the patient. Examples include not confronting the therapy patient who often arrives late for, or misses, his appointments because the behavior is ascribed to "cultural factors" or missing observable cues of depression (e.g., restricted affect, poor eye contact) because it is "culturally congruent." These cultural considerations are clinical hypotheses to be tested. Moreover, they fall within the purview of psychiatric clinical ethics (see Chapters 1, 2, and 6) because of the heightened responsibility of mental health providers to be attuned to the concerns and experiences of patients in the context of serving their health and well-being. Beyond this, mental health providers have a special responsibility to be self-observing in the therapeutic interaction and, therefore, to monitor their own assumptions about cultural influences on patient care.

Limited Access to Clinical Care, Mental Health, and Ethics Resources

Resource limitations generate numerous ethical problems for small-community clinicians. Health care access obstacles include resources limitations in the continuum of services, relative effectiveness of services, actual use of services, willingness to use services, and ability to use services. Many rural areas, for example, do not have emergency, urgent care, or specialty care facilities. Roughly 7% of rural counties in the United States have no physicians at all, and a majority of rural counties lack psychiatric, pediatric, obstetric, and other doctoral-level specialist care (Braden and Beauregard 1994). In a study of 160 caregivers in Alaska and New Mexico, clinicians in smaller communities (population less than 2,500) indicated a lack of health care resources and an inability to find personal health care (Roberts et al. 2003). Rural nurses have expanded roles and responsibilities, with greater autonomy, the need for extensive knowledge, but with less training and fewer resources than urban nurses. Nurses and nursing assistants, physicians' assistants, social workers and aides, and "deputized" local citizens often serve as caregivers in small communities. In frontier villages in Alaska, Maine, and Appalachia, a patient's entire treatment team may consist of family members who have no training and little support from care providers. Problems related both to professional responsibility and personal exhaustion commonly arise when "keeping watch" over suicidal, manic, or psychotic patients under such circumstances.

Many small communities also do not have hospitals or hospital-based supports, including specialty consultants who can help improve clinical standards of care. Relative effectiveness of care may be limited by poor multidisciplinary care services, for example, leading to insufficient physical and psychological therapies and/or late detection of illness. Willingness to pursue and accept care and the actual use of services may be affected by a wide variety of factors, such as the ethnicity and cultural background of the care providers, perceived quality of past treatment, the time of year (e.g., harvest season), the language(s) spoken in the clinic, and attitudinal factors such as the clinician's acceptance of alternative healing practices (Henderson et al. 1997). Rural patients have been found to be twice as likely as urban patients to have to travel for over 30 minutes to reach their usual source of health care. Rural clinics may also be less well equipped than urban centers to handle the special requirements of disabled patients. Rural clinicians may hesitate to send patients far from home for serious medical conditions because of the absence of supports in these distant cities. Their patients may not have transportation or money for such outside care. These rural health care attributes affect patients' ability to use services. Overall, access considerations have become more severe as managed care companies and capitated care systems have entered rural areas (Stout 1998). Many similar problems are mirrored in urban areas with distinct subpopulations, such as immigrants or religious groups. In response to such resource limitations, clinicians may be forced to provide care outside of their usual areas of expertise, a practice that poses risk for both clinical and ethical errors. Greater attention to care issues in small communities or subcommunities in large urban areas is thus critical in terms of the fair distribution of medical resources, a key social justice issue in this country.

As described in Chapters 1, 2, and 4, ethically sound care in complex cases often entails a consultative process—with a bioethics committee, an ethics or legal expert, or a knowledgeable colleague. Ethics review processes, both formal and informal, are not readily available in many small-community situations, however. Ethics committees do not exist in most small-town hospitals and clinics, and when they do, they grapple with the same overlapping-role and role-conflict issues, confidentiality problems, and other dilemmas of rural providers. Ethics experts and specialist colleagues, peers, and supervisors may not always be available in isolated areas. Even in urban small communities, outside consultants may not appreciate the subtleties of the patient's immediately surrounding culture and expectations or the small-community clinician's special conflicts.

Clinicians in these areas often feel that sources of information on identifying and resolving clinical ethical dilemmas (e.g., bioethics literature, forensic textbooks, professional ethics codes) are so "out of touch" or incongruent with the realities of the small-community context that they are unhelpful (Niemira 1988). Because of these problems, small-community clinicians sometimes develop their own guidelines for resolving ethical problems. Because these innovative "solutions" may deviate from national standards, these factors place the small-community practitioner at risk for true ethical misjudgments as well as complaints of perceived misconduct (Turner et al. 1996). In a study of 510 Kansas physicians' strategies for safeguarding patient confidentiality, nearly half of the small-community physicians reported that friends or family members accounted for a significant proportion of their patients. In contrast, these two issues of patient confidentiality and appropriate boundary-setting affected only 13% of the physicians serving larger communities. Approaches used by survey respondents to protect patient confidentiality were speaking with office personnel regarding the importance of confidentiality of the specific patient (88% of respondents), omitting certain details from the official medical record (69%), recording the importance of confidentiality in the chart (46%), omitting certain details from insurance forms (37%), neglecting to perform a required notification of local public health officials (21%), and purposeful misrepresentation of details in the medical record (6%) or insurance forms (5%) (Ullom-Minnich and Kallail 1993). This study shows how the size of a community may influence confidentiality practice patterns, including behaviors that are not acceptable by formal ethics and clinical practice standards. Consequently, greater availability of ethics resources and special efforts to address the dilemmas encountered by small-community clinicians may help bring about problem-solving strategies that may differ with approaches in other communities but do not violate basic ethics principles and professional values held more widely throughout medicine.

Stresses of Small-Community Caregivers

Although small-community clinicians are highly valued individuals, they experience unique stresses as a consequence of their overlapping roles, their rigorous daily work responsibilities in the absence of adequate support and expertise, and their personal and professional isolation. Relentless visibility and limited time and health care access may be poorly appreciated obstacles to personal self-care of rural clinicians. Exhaustion, "burnout," cynicism, and impairment are predictable outcomes of such stresses. These factors, in turn, may contribute to the known problems of short tenure and frequent relocation of rural practitioners. Positive protective forces such as community support, hardiness, and affirmation in one's professional role may help mitigate these pressures. Nevertheless, from an ethics perspective, these context-driven stresses may narrow the repertoire of problem-solving approaches that a clinician may draw upon in comparison with other situations that have more opportunities for reflection, for management of stress, and for expert supervision and consultation.

■ CONSTRUCTIVE APPROACHES

Small-community clinicians are highly dedicated individuals—people who undertake the special challenges of their situation, often in fulfillment of deeply held personal and professional values. Small-community practitioners often feel a special commitment to promoting the processes of health and recovery seen throughout their communities. These thoughtful clinicians continually create constructive approaches to the therapeutic relationship dilemmas, problems of limited resources, stresses, and moral binds they experience.

Positive strategies for dealing with ethical dilemmas in small-community settings are several. First, maintaining relationships with colleagues in other areas will help to lessen the sense of isolation and disconnection from the profession. This is very important, because colleagues with clinical, legal, or ethics expertise (e.g., on hospital-based ethics committees) are often not available to provide information, guidance, or support for small-community care providers. Participating in postgraduate and continuing-education activities is also valuable in terms of learning about clinical and ethical standards of care. Building a network of multidisciplinary experts through innovative technology such as the Internet and telemedicine will allow for consultation or referral on difficult cases. In this process, seeking to educate colleagues on a regional and national level about the challenges of small-community care is critically important. Active involvement with consumer groups, professional organizations, local leaders, and agency representatives may help to bring attention and resources to underserved communities. Moreover, advocating for health service resources and suggesting adaptive and appropriate revisions of extant ethics guidelines are additional steps that can be taken to help future clinicians who serve in small-community settings. Increasing awareness of these issues will help these practitioners to deal with the distress and aloneness they may undergo in relation to the ethical complexities inherent to their situation.

Second, when it is necessary to take actions that would appear to differ from national ethics standards, it is important to think through the reasons and implications of this choice from an ethical perspective. Further, it is optimal to take several steps to ensure that patients are sufficiently safeguarded. For instance, in an interdependent frontier community, accepting gifts or bartering for services may be fundamental to the shared life and practices of the community. Even so, there may be gifts that are too large to accept ethically or individuals from whom services and resources should not be traded because of the specific unequal nature of the professional–patient relationship. In such situations where urban ethics rules and guidelines are not readily applied, the processes by which the rural clinician seeks to act ethically gain immense importance. Comparing one's practices with those of other rural and frontier clinicians, seeking consultation from trusted colleagues, developing written clinic policies, documenting decisions, and accurately disclosing what one has chosen to do are important process steps that ethical clinicians can employ.

Third, taking proactive steps to address the interconnected issues of overlapping roles and confidentiality is very important for small-community clinicians. Talking with office staff and multidisciplinary team members about the ethical problems associated with personal and professional relationships in small communities, for instance, is a crucial measure employed by many wise rural clinicians. In this process, it is important to follow up on any "leaks" or "slips" of patient information that may occur so that the message of protecting patients is made unambiguously. Creating "backup" arrangements so that members of the clinical care team may excuse themselves from sensitive cases such as family members, without leaving their colleagues "in the lurch," is important for patients and colleagues. At times, it may be necessary to refer patients to receive care in neighboring communities. Over time, it may be possible to build collaborative networks of reciprocal care across communities to help in such situations. Conscientious clinicians will also remain attentive to the impact of overlapping roles on the patient perspective—how patients may feel apprehensive about the conflicts associated with these roles and how these conflicts may create barriers to pursuing or accepting care. Talking through the challenges of overlapping relationships with patients is also constructive. Efforts to separate personal and professional roles to whatever extent is possible will help with these conflicts. Clinicians may wish to address their patients on a first-name basis at the post office or the ball park, for instance, but choose to talk with their patients on a more formal basis as "Mrs. Jones" or "Mr. McDonald" at the clinic.

Efforts to address confidentiality in small communities ranging from the medical school student health clinic to a Native American pueblo include careful confidentiality "routines" such as keeping computer screens and private records out of sight, conducting telephone conversations (e.g., to the pharmacy, to a consulting clinician) behind closed doors, maintaining separate "shadow" charts when necessary, and encoding patient material in both written charts and computer databases. It is helpful when medical and psychiatric or psychological services are both available through a single clinic so that the stigma associated with the need for mental health care is minimized.

Fourth, the clinician should enlist the help of leaders in the community in building effective strategies for dealing with the specific cultural issues they face. Clinicians who are new to a community should expect a period of intensive learning and testing initially. Clinicians who seek to understand their community's history and their patients' authentic concerns will often be well accepted, if only from necessity, even if the clinicians come from very different personal backgrounds than those of their patients. Indeed, it is not necessary to "blend in" or to lose one's own identity in order to be an effective caregiver. It is nevertheless essential to have a sense of one's own cultural beliefs and to reflect upon their influence in the clinician–patient relationship. Fidelity to the well-being of the patient in the context of the patient's own background and value system is often the key to this process. Consequently, small-community clinicians will need to remain flexible—but to a limit. For instance, if the clinician is asked, implicitly or explicitly, to make choices that vary greatly from other communities' standards, it will be important for the clinician to obtain supervision and support from colleagues. When making decisions that are at odds with the preferences of the community, it will be important to communicate the values and restrictions that underlie these decisions. Framing the decisions as reflections of clinical necessity or as manifestations of professional integrity will at least help the community to understand what is happening. Moreover, addressing clinical mistakes in a culturally congruent manner will do much to establish the credibility of the small-community practitioner. Finally, for clinicians who have grown up in or practiced for a long time in a particular community, it will be necessary to think through and periodically reconsider their assumptions about cultural expectations, which may be rapidly evolving given the growing influence of urban values through new media and communication avenues (e.g., cable television, the Internet, satellite-based telephone services). In this context, small-community practitioners will also need to be mindful of the cultural significance of their clinical role for their patients by virtue of their ethnicity, gender, age, urban training and education, community status, and other personal attributes.

Finally, personal self-care is an important professional task for small-community clinicians. Identifying and minimizing career-related stresses, pursuing ways of reducing role conflicts, balancing one's caseload and pacing one's practice patterns, taking vacations, developing adequate "backup" coverage approaches, obtaining personal health care such as annual physical examinations, and other activities are crucial. These efforts will help the practitioner to be emotionally and physically healthy and to remain able to do the hard work of small-community care.

Case Scenarios

A school counselor in a very small community in Idaho develops a serious problem with alcohol. The nearest treatment center is 200 miles away.

A woman goes to see the physician assistant because she has felt suicidal. The receptionist is her next-door neighbor.

The only therapist in an Alaskan village must purchase all of his essential goods from patients or family members of patients.

A scientist working for a government laboratory is afraid to seek treatment for a recurring cocaine problem. He informally asks the occupational health physician, whom he trusts, for the name of a psychiatrist. Fearful of losing his security clearance, he asks that the occupational health physician make no mention of his request to anyone and that the physician not document the referral in his records.

The only doctor in a remote community believes that one of his patients is developing postpartum psychosis. Because he does not feel competent to treat her, he calls the nearest university medical center to see if he can arrange a consultation.

■ REFERENCES

Braden J, Beauregard K: Health status and access to care of rural and urban populations. National Medical Expenditure Survey Research Findings 18 (AHCPR Publ No. 94-0031). Rockville, MD, Agency for Health Care Policy and Research, 1994

Henderson G, King NMP, Strauss RP, et al. (eds): The Social Medicine Reader. Durham, NC, Duke University Press, 1997

Niemira DA: Grassroots grappling: ethics committees at rural hospitals. Ann Intern Med 109:981–983, 1988

Perkins DV, Hudson BL, Gray DM, et al: Decisions and justifications by community mental health providers about hypothetical ethical dilemmas. Psychiatr Serv 49:1317–1322, 1998

Roberts LW, Monaghan-Geernaert P, Battaglia J, Warner TD: Personal health care attitudes of rural clinicians: a preliminary study of 127 multi-disciplinary health care providers in Alaska and New Mexico. Rural Mental Health 28(1), 2003

Simon RI: Treatment boundary violations: clinical, ethical, and legal considerations. Bull Am Acad Psychiatry Law 20:269–288, 1992

Simon RI, Williams IC: Maintaining treatment boundaries in small communities and rural areas. Psychiatr Serv 50:1440–1446, 1999

Stout M: Impact of Medicaid managed mental health care on delivery of services in a rural state: an AMI perspective. Psychiatr Serv 49:961–963, 1998

Turner LN, Marquis K, Burman ME: Rural nurse practitioners: perceptions of ethical dilemmas. J Am Acad Nurse Pract 8:269–274, 1996

Ullom-Minnich PD, Kallail KJ: Physicians' strategies for safeguarding confidentiality: the influence of community and practice characteristics. J Fam Pract 37:445–448, 1993

11

CARING FOR PEOPLE AT END OF LIFE

The inevitability of death is one of the central features of existence. This is so for all living things, but human beings uniquely have the ability to reflect on this reality. Even so, the certainty of death is a truth that we tend not to keep in consciousness, to repress, forget, or even to deny. Ensuring that explicit conversations about end-of-life care occur is an important task for all clinicians in our society, especially given the impact of modern technologies and health care systems on the occurrence and process of death.

From a mental health perspective, psychological suffering prior to death may be immense, and psychiatric disorders may distort decisions and processes in the dying process. Death may trigger significant psychiatric symptoms among grieving loved ones. Psychiatrists, psychologists, nurses, therapists, counselors, and other mental health caregivers may indeed have particularly important roles in preparing patients for death, safeguarding dying persons, and helping those who grieve.

■ SIX DOMAINS FOR CAREFUL ATTENTION

Mental health clinicians may find it valuable to organize their thinking about end-of-life care for their patients in relation to six domains (Table 11–1): diagnosis, comfort, capacity, clarity, controversy, and collaboration.

TABLE 11–1.	**Six domains for consideration by mental health clinicians in end-of-life care**
Diagnosis	What is the dying person's medical condition? What is the anticipated course of the illness? Are there features of the illness that will cause physical pain, psychiatric and/or cognitive disturbances, or specific forms of disability? Does the dying person have evidence of a psychiatric disorder, such as delirium, major depression, or anxiety? Has appropriate treatment been initiated?
Comfort	Have diligent efforts to assess the physical and psychological pain been undertaken? What comfort measures are in place and are planned? Does the dying person understand what pain control measures are in his or her direct control? Have clear approaches to "stepping up" the pain control been discussed, so that the patient can request this?
Capacity	What is the decisional capacity of the dying person? What is the voluntarism capacity of the dying person? Has every reasonable effort been made to improve the patient's capacities when he or she is making key treatment decisions (e.g., through careful efforts to address physical pain, to minimize use of unnecessary psychotropic medications)?
Clarity	Are the patient's values and wishes clear regarding end-of-life care? Is there appropriate documentation to assist all clinicians and family members involved in the care of the patient?
Controversy	Have the tough issues been addressed with the patient and his or her loved ones? Are the views of the patient, of key decision makers (e.g., family members), and of other individuals involved (e.g., the clinical care team, community members) known? If there are sources of controversy, have these been addressed carefully, with specific roles, boundaries, and decision-making processes and options clearly laid out?

TABLE 11–1.	**Six domains for consideration by mental health clinicians in end-of-life care** *(continued)*
Collaboration	For the benefit of the dying person, have all of the people—loved ones, multidisciplinary clinicians, community members—been appropriately included? Do other people or resources need to be invited in to help the patient?

Diagnosis

It is crucial that the mental health clinician understand key aspects of the dying person's physical illness and remain vigilant for signs of a psychiatric disorder, which may greatly affect the patient's care and decision making. The clinician should have a working understanding of the nature and course of the patient's medical condition. To provide optimal care, several questions should be clear in the clinician's mind. For example, what is the anticipated course of the illness? Are there features of the illness that will cause physical pain, psychiatric and/or cognitive disturbances, or specific forms of disability? For instance, if the illness is a form of cancer, is it especially likely to cause physical pain? To spread quickly or slowly? Is it locally invasive, or does it spread to distant sites, including the brain which may affect the person's cognitive and emotional functioning? Does the dying person have evidence of a psychiatric disorder, such as delirium, major depression, anxiety, or psychosis? Have causes of symptoms—ranging from adjustment issues, disease-related issues, adverse effects of medications, and preexisting illnesses—been carefully established? Is the main caregiver aware of the potential impact of the medical condition on the psychological well-being and the psychiatric status of the patient? Has appropriate treatment been initiated for the medical condition or for primary or secondary psychiatric processes that coexist?

Comfort

Beyond accurate diagnosis and appropriate treatment, comfort is an imperative in caring for dying persons. Pain is what many fear most about the dying process. Making every effort to help the person have some control over pain is a positive contribution to the care of a dying patient. Toward this goal, physical and psychological pain should be carefully assessed, using both subjective and objective measures, and then clearly documented for all clinicians involved in the care of the patient. This evaluation may include formal tools, such as measures of quality of life (Appendix A at the end of this chapter presents an example of such a tool). A number of comfort measures should be planned and put in place for the future care of the patient. More than this, however, the patient should understand these measures and the extent to which they are in his or her direct control. Specific steps to facilitate communication about the need for enhanced treatment for pain should be addressed early and remembered explicitly together in the care of the dying person.

The mental health clinician has a special role in tracking the internal experience of the dying person. In one patient, this may mean helping to dismantle barriers to requesting help and pain medications. For another patient, it may mean working through loss, anger, and existential issues. For yet another patient, it may mean helping the clinicians to see the culturally sanctioned comforts valued and needed by the patient. The mental health clinician should remain attentive to psychological, cultural, and social issues from the perspective of the patient. Ultimately this means that the mental health caregiver serves as both an advocate and a healer in seeking and providing comfort for dying persons.

Capacity

Formally assessing decisional capacity in the context of end-of-life care is a vital role of consultation-liaison and general adult psychiatrists, nurse specialists, primary care physicians, and psychologists with specialized interests in this area. Chapter 4 provides a detailed discussion of the systematic assessment of decisional and voluntarism capacities. Therapists and counselors working with dying persons will also need some sense of patients' strengths and deficits, their ability to make crucial clinical care decisions, and when to talk with the main clinical team about concerns about their changing status.

In thinking about the care of a dying person, the mental health clinicians ideally will ask a series of questions: What is the set of overall strengths and deficits of the patient? What is the patient's decisional capacity, as assessed along the four dimensions of communication, understanding, reasoning, and appreciation? What is the patient's capacity for voluntarism, as assessed along the four dimensions of developmental, illness-related, psychological and cultural, and contextual factors? Has every reasonable effort been made to improve the patient's capacity when he or she is making key treatment decisions? This includes a wide set of activities, such as careful efforts to diagnose and treat overlooked psychiatric conditions; to relieve physical pain; to address grief and psychological pain; to include family, spiritual, and/or culturally appropriate supports; and to minimize use of unnecessary psychotropic medications.

Clarity

As clinicians committed to understanding the experiences and the ability of our patients to make meaning, mental health caregivers have a special responsibility to ensure that the dying person's values and wishes are clarified regarding end-of-life care. Some dying persons will have thought a great deal about these issues and will have a sophisticated understanding of the kinds of decisions required in modern medical situations. Some other patients will not, for many reasons that relate to psychological defenses and emotional distress to educational level and geographic isolation. Tools such as the values history (see Appendix B at the end of this chapter) and the spiritual history (Table 11–2) are excellent resources for facilitating discussions of these issues with patients, their families, and their caregivers. This allows the voice and preferences of the dying person to be identified and honored, not presumed or usurped. It allows their dignity and personhood to be preserved in the face of great fear and loss. Toward this aim, it is also crucial to ensure that appropriate

---

TABLE 11–2. **Illustrative questions to ask in taking a spiritual history**

F—Faith and belief

"Do you consider yourself spiritual or religious?" or *"Do you have spiritual beliefs that help you cope with stress?"* If the patient responds "no," the physician might ask, *"What gives your life meaning?"* Sometimes patients respond with answers such as family, career, or nature.

I—Importance

"What importance does your faith or belief have in your life? Have your beliefs influenced how you take care of yourself in this illness? What role do your beliefs play in regaining your health?"

C—Community

"Are you a part of a spiritual or religious community? Is this a support for you? Is there a group of people you really love or who are important to you?" Communities such as churches, temples, and mosques or a group of like-minded friends can serve as strong support systems for some patients.

A—Address in care

"How would you like me, your health care provider, to address these issues in your health care?"

Source.   Adapted from Puchalski and Romer 2000.

---

documentation of the patient's values and preferences exists and is available to assist all clinicians and family members involved in the care of the patient. With the permission of the patient, clinical advance directives and other formal legal documents should be prepared, and multiple copies should be distributed to all appropriate clinicians, health care facilities, and family members.

Controversy

The experiences of loss are often accompanied by controversy and by controversial decision making, and dying is no exception. The mental health clinician can help anticipate the complex, controversial issues that may arise so that they may be acknowledged and worked on explicitly, respectfully, and with appropriate "rules of engagement." Every practicing physician has experienced a situation where, just after a constructive, supportive plan has been developed to provide care for a dying person, a late-arriving sibling, an estranged spouse, a beloved child who has been out of the country, or a nephew with aspirations for an inheritance—who has not been involved in the therapeutic planning process—will cry "wait, how can you do this to him?!" In part motivated by fear of litigation, the process comes to a halt, and the positive work of supporting the dying patient can come completely undone. Intensive, prospective efforts to identify key individuals involved, immediately or more remotely, in the patient's life and to identify potential areas of disagreement or controversy are extraordinarily helpful in this process. It is important to note that the personal views of the mental health clinician figure into this as well, and considerable self-understanding of one's own preferences (and biases) regarding palliative care and difficult topics such as rational suicide, assisted death, and euthanasia is essential. The clinician therefore should ask the following questions: Have the tough issues been addressed with the patient and loved ones? Are the views of the patient, of key decision makers (e.g., family members), and of other individuals involved (e.g., the clinical care team, community members) known? If there are sources of controversy, have these been addressed carefully, with specific roles, boundaries, and decision-making processes and options clearly laid out?

Collaboration

The dying person's needs should be the ultimate consideration. It is important for the mental health clinician to determine whether consultation with other people—including loved ones; clinicians from other disciplines; attorneys; rabbis, priests, or other spiritual leaders; and community members—should be pursued for the benefit of the dying person. It may help to mobilize other resources as well, such as palliative care experts and hospice clinicians.

■ EMERGENT ETHICAL QUESTIONS IN END-OF-LIFE CARE

Beyond these six domains of immediate importance to mental health clinicians in providing end-of-life care is the societal context in which that care is provided. Modern technology has altered how we understand death—what it is and when it occurs. The recognition that there could be such a thing as a "good death" has been a constant tension throughout the history of medicine. The fourth paragraph of the Hippocratic Oath admonishes physicians to "neither give a deadly drug to anybody if asked for it, nor make a suggestion to this effect." Most states have passed legislation focusing on "death with dignity." Physicians can make things better for patients, can alleviate suffering and sometimes cure disease, and can forestall—but not overcome—death. This said, the international debate on the ethical acceptability of assisted death practices—encompassing physician-assisted suicide and euthanasia—is intense, and people of goodwill exist on all sides of these controversial issues.

Many psychiatrists, including one of the authors (LWR), have expressed concern about the emergence of assisted death practices in light of what is understood about the clinical phenomena of suicide and in light of important empirical work on attitudes toward assisted death practices. As described in Chapter 5, as many as 95% of individuals who commit suicide have preexisting and often treatable mental illnesses (Hendin and Klerman 1993). Psychiatric diseases such as depression and delirium and their symptoms and signs—such as negative cognitive distortions, hopelessness, difficulty with concentration, and despair—may greatly influence a request for assisted death, just as it has been shown that severe, treatable physical pain will prompt this same request in oncology settings (Roberts et al. 1997). Psychiatrists are also very cognizant of the complexities of obtaining informed consent for major health care decisions in the context of very serious or terminal illness and of how vulnerable patients with great suffering can be. Just as ethical palliative care is based on diagnosing and addressing sources of suffering, ethical mental health care at end of life has the same imperatives.

Intriguing empirical work suggests the importance of these issues. Studies of people with advanced cancer reveal that the preference for assisted death is not common, although, importantly, it is an accurate marker of treatable major depression (Emanuel et al. 1996). Interest in assisted death practices as expressed by 378 persons with HIV in another study was determined by lack of emotional support, by psychological distress, and by symptoms of mental illness rather than physical illness determinants (Breitbart et al. 1996). In a classic study of elderly psychiatric inpatients, the most severely depressed and hopeless patients overestimated the risks and underestimated the benefits of medical care at end of life (Ganzini et al. 1994). With appropriate mental health treatment, these beliefs reversed, and the patients changed their end-of-life care preferences to allow for more intensive therapeutic interventions. A series of studies performed by one of the authors (LWR) with colleagues suggested that as medical students, residents, and physicians advance through training, their acceptance of assisted death practices decreases and that psychiatrists are significantly less supportive of assisted suicide and euthanasia than are physicians in other specialty areas (Roberts 1997). This work also indicated that clinicians are more comfortable with the performance of assisted death by others, although they themselves are unwilling to engage in these activities. This finding has important implications related to moral agency within the clinical professions.

Debates about the rights and wrongs of end-of-life issues travel from the courts to the bedside and back to the courts and legislatures. But death, clearly, is distinctly human and distinctly personal in a manner that is not captured by these busy, complex, psychologically distant events. End-of-life conversations touch on the most inner subjective aspects of the meaning of life and death. Mental health clinicians who can help keep this focus will do much to serve their dying patients.

Case Scenarios

An 80-year-old retired technician with metastatic lung cancer refuses further chemotherapy because, he says, "there is nothing it can fix." His children become very upset and demand that he receive psychiatric treatment for depression.

A 67-year-old man career military officer whose wife has advanced Alzheimer's disease is diagnosed with colon cancer. He tells his son that he thinks it would be better if "both of us were out of the way."

Before undergoing a quadruple bypass, a very active 72-year-old woman fills out an advance directive assigning power of attorney for health care to her husband.

A 54-year-old woman with progressive multiple sclerosis is wheelchair bound and unable to perform any tasks of daily living for herself. She asks the psychiatrists treating her for depression if he could arrange to give her "too many sleeping pills."

A 75-year-old farmer who is filling out an advance directive indicates that he does not want to "depend on any machines."

■ REFERENCES

Breitbart W, Rosenfeld BD, Passik SD: Interest in physician-assisted suicide among ambulatory HIV-infected patients [see comments]. Am J Psychiatry 153:238–242, 1996

Emanuel EJ, Fairclough DL, Daniels ER, et al: Euthanasia and physician-assisted suicide: attitudes and experiences of oncology patients, oncologists, and the public. Lancet 347:1805–1810, 1996

Ganzini L, Lee MA, Heintz RT, et al: The effect of depression treatment on elderly patients' preferences for life-sustaining medical therapy [see comments]. Am J Psychiatry 151:1631–1636, 1994

Hendin H, Klerman GL: Physician-assisted suicide: the dangers of legalization. Am J Psychiatry 150:143–145, 1993

Puchalski CM, Romer AL: Taking a spiritual history allows clinicians to understand patients more fully. Journal of Palliative Medicine 3:129–137, 2000

Roberts LW: Sequential assessment of medical student competence with respect to professional attitudes, values, and ethics. Subcommittee on Professional Attitudes and Values, Student Progress Assessment. Acad Med 72:428–429, 1997

Roberts LW, Muskin PR, Warner TD, et al: Attitudes of consultation-liaison psychiatrists toward physician- assisted death practices. Psychosomatics 38:459–471, 1997

Appendix A

MISSOULA–VITAS
QUALITY OF LIFE INDEX™

APPENDIX A. **Missoula–VITAS Quality of Life Index™ V-15**

INSTRUCTIONS: Indicate the extent to which you agree or disagree with the following statements by marking in one of the boxes below the question. For items with two statements, indicate agreements with one or the other or if they are equally true, choose "Neutral." If you make a mistake or change your mind, place an X through the wrong answer and mark the box indicating your correct answer.

Patient's Name: _____ Today's Date: _____

GLOBAL

How would you rate your overall quality of life?

❑	❑	❑	❑	❑
Worse Possible	Poor	Fair	Good	Best Possible

SYMPTOMS

1. I feel sick all the time.

❑	❑	❑	❑	❑
Agree Strongly	Agree	Neutral	Disagree	Disagree Strongly

2. I am satisfied with current control of my symptoms.

❑	❑	❑	❑	❑
Agree Strongly	Agree	Neutral	Disagree	Disagree Strongly

APPENDIX A.   **Missoula–VITAS Quality of Life Index™ V-15** *(continued)*

3. Despite physical discomfort, in general I can enjoy my days.

OR

Physical discomfort overshadows any opportunity for enjoyment.

Agree Strongly	Agree	Neutral	Disagree	Disagree Strongly
❑	❑	❑	❑	❑

4. I am still able to do many of the things I like to do.

OR

I am no longer able to do many of the things I like to do.

Agree Strongly	Agree	Neutral	Disagree	Disagree Strongly
❑	❑	❑	❑	❑

5. I accept the fact that I cannot do many of the things I used to do.

OR

I am disappointed that I cannot do many of the things I used to do.

Agree Strongly	Agree	Neutral	Disagree	Disagree Strongly
❑	❑	❑	❑	❑

6. My contentment with life depends upon being active and being independent in my personal care.

Agree Strongly	Agree	Neutral	Disagree	Disagree Strongly
❑	❑	❑	❑	❑

APPENDIX A.   Missoula–VITAS Quality of Life Index™ V-15 *(continued)*

INTERPERSONAL

7. I have recently been able to say important things to the people close to me.

Agree Strongly	Agree	Neutral	Disagree	Disagree Strongly
❏	❏	❏	❏	❏

8. At present, I spend as much time as I want to with family and friends.

Agree Strongly	Agree	Neutral	Disagree	Disagree Strongly
❏	❏	❏	❏	❏

9. It is important to me to have close personal relationships.

Agree Strongly	Agree	Neutral	Disagree	Disagree Strongly
❏	❏	❏	❏	❏

WELL-BEING

10. My affairs are in order; I could die today with a clear mind.
OR
My affairs are not in order; I am worried that many things are unresolved.

Agree Strongly	Agree	Neutral	Disagree	Disagree Strongly
❏	❏	❏	❏	❏

11. I am more satisfied with myself as a person now than I was before my illness.

Agree Strongly	Agree	Neutral	Disagree	Disagree Strongly
❏	❏	❏	❏	❏

APPENDIX A. **Missoula–VITAS Quality of Life Index™ V-15** *(continued)*

12. It is important to me to be at peace with myself.

Agree Strongly	Agree	Neutral	Disagree	Disagree Strongly
□	□	□	□	□

TRANSCENDENT

13. I have a better sense of meaning in my life now than I have had in the past.

OR

I have less of a sense of meaning in my life now than I have had in the past.

Agree Strongly	Agree	Neutral	Disagree	Disagree Strongly
□	□	□	□	□

14. Life has become more precious to me; every day is a gift.

OR

Life has lost all value for me; every day is a burden.

Agree Strongly	Agree	Neutral	Disagree	Disagree Strongly
□	□	□	□	□

15. It is important to me to feel that my life has meaning.

Agree Strongly	Agree	Neutral	Disagree	Disagree Strongly
□	□	□	□	□

Source. Copyright 1998–2001, VITAS Healthcare Corporation, Miami, FL, and Ira R. Byock, M.D., Missoula, MT. Do not reproduce without permission.

Appendix B

VALUES HISTORY FORM

NAME: _____ _____ DATE: _____

If someone assisted you in completing this form, please fill in his or her
  name, address, and relationship to you.

    Name:

    Address:

    Relationship:

Overall attitude toward life and health

What would you like to say about your overall attitude toward life to
  someone reading this document?

What goals do you have for the future?

How satisfied are you with what you have achieved in your life?

What, for you, makes life worth living?

What do you fear most? What frightens or upsets you?

What activities do you enjoy (e.g., hobbies, watching TV)?

How would you describe your current state of health?

If you currently have any health problems or disabilities, how do they
  affect...

    You?

    Your family?

    Your work?

    Your ability to function?

If you have health problems or disabilities, how do you feel about them?
  What would you like others (family, friends, doctors) to know about this?

Do you have difficulty getting through the day with activities such as...

    Eating?

    Preparing food?

    Sleeping?

    Dressing, bathing, etc.?

What would you like to say about your general health to someone reading
  this document?

APPENDIX B. **Values History Form** *(continued)*

Personal relationships

What role do family and friends play in your life?

How do you expect friends, family, and others to support your decisions regarding medical treatment you may need now or in the future?

Have you made any arrangements for family or friends to make medical treatment decisions on your behalf? If so, who has agreed to make decisions for you and in what circumstances?

What general comments would you like to make about the personal relationships in your life?

Thoughts about independence and self-sufficiency

How does independence or dependence affect your life?

If you were to experience decreased physical and mental abilities, how would that affect your attitude toward independence and self-sufficiency?

If your current physical or mental health gets worse, how would you feel?

Living environment

Have you lived alone or with others over the past 10 years?

How comfortable have you been in your surroundings? How might illness, disability, or age affect this?

What general comments would you like to make about your surroundings?

Religious background and beliefs

What is your spiritual/religious background?

How do your beliefs affect your feelings toward serious, chronic, or terminal illness?

How does your faith community, church, or synagogue support you?

What general comments would you like to make about your beliefs?

Relationships with doctors and other health caregivers

How do you relate to your doctors? Please comment on: trust, decision making, time for satisfactory communication, respectful treatment.

How do you feel about other caregivers, including nurses, therapists, chaplains, social workers, etc.?

What else would you like to say about doctors and other caregivers?

Thoughts about illness, dying, and death

What general comments would you like to make about illness, dying, and death?

What will be important to you when you are dying (e.g., physical comfort, no pain, family members present)?

Where would you prefer to die?

How do you feel about the use of life-sustaining measures if you were…

Suffering from an irreversible chronic illness (e.g., Alzheimer's disease)?

Terminally ill?

In a permanent coma?

What general comments would you like to make about medical treatment?

Finances

What general comments would you like to make about your finances and the cost of health care?

What are your feelings about having enough money to provide for your care?

Funeral plans

What general comments would you like to make about your funeral and burial or cremation?

Have you made your funeral arrangements? If so, with whom?

Optional questions

How would you like your obituary (announcement of your death) to read?

Write yourself a brief eulogy (a statement about yourself to be read at your funeral).

What would you like to say to someone reading this Values History Form?

Legal documents

Which of the following legal documents about health care decisions have you signed? (Each state has its own special form; feel free to add yours to this list.)

- **An advance directive for health care for your state?** Yes ___ No ___
    Where and with whom can it be found?
    Name:
    Address:
    Phone:
- **A living will?** Yes ___ No ___
    Where and with whom can it be found?
    Name:
    Address:
    Phone:

APPENDIX B.   **Values History Form** *(continued)*

- **A durable power of attorney for health care decisions?** Yes ___ No ___

    Where and with whom can it be found?

    Name:

    Address:

    Phone:

- **A health care proxy?** Yes ___ No ___

    Where and with whom can it be found?

    Name:

    Address:

    Phone:

Source.   Reprinted from Gibson JM, Lambert P, Nathanson P: "The Values History: An Innovation in Surrogate Medical Decision-Making." *Law, Medicine, and Health Care* 18(3):202–212, 1990. Used with permission.

ETHICAL ISSUES IN
PSYCHIATRIC GENETICS

With Cynthia M.A. Geppert, M.D., Ph.D.

Almost every day, the media announces a new genetic break-through. Many of these stories report discoveries relating to the genetics of mental illness that offer new hope for patients and families with serious psychiatric disorders. This genetic revolution also raises unprecedented ethical concerns. Although the heritability of mental illness has been recognized for hundreds of years, the extraordinary progress of molecular biology and the Human Genome Project together have introduced a new complexity and uncertainty into key safeguards, such as informed consent and confidentiality, and have generated unique ethical, legal, religious, and social dilemmas.

Whereas most psychiatric genetic work is now conducted in a research context, the coming years will see the translation of this science to the offices of clinical psychiatrists, neurologists, and some primary care clinicians. Psychiatric genetics may involve testing asymptomatic individuals with a predisposition to mental illness, persons who potentially carry susceptibility genes for psychiatric disorders, and mentally ill individuals with genetic variants or markers that might pertain to the efficacy and safety of medications—that is, the new field of pharmacogenetics. One day in the not-too-distant future, gene therapy for mental disorders may be a part of psychiatric treatment. Thus, it is important for practitioners to understand the fundamental ethics of informed consent and confidentiality and considerations of justice that surround psychiatric genetics.

■ THE NATURE OF GENETIC INFORMATION

Genetic information is health information with subtle differences that are of particular ethical significance for mental illness. Psychiatric genetic information is 1) complex, 2) probabilistic, 3) familial, and 4) existential. With the exception of Huntington's disease and several variants of familial Alzheimer's disease, every major neuropsychiatric disorder is thought to be a complex disorder. A complex genetic disorder is the result not of a single gene, but of several genes interacting with each other and with the environment. The recent National Institute of Mental Health Workgroup established a substantial complex genetic component to nearly every Axis I disorder, but as of this writing, no gene has been identified as causative of major mental illnesses such as bipolar disorder or schizophrenia (National Institute of Mental Health Genetics Workgroup 1997).

■ INFORMED CONSENT IN PSYCHIATRIC GENETICS

The complex nature of psychiatric disorders means that even when genes are identified as involved in the development of psychiatric disorders, possession of these genes confers only a risk or probability, not a certainty, that an individual or a family member will develop a psychiatric condition. A person who has several members of his family diagnosed with schizophrenia clearly has a greater vulnerability than a member of the general population. However, family history does not unalterably dictate the development of a disorder, nor does it determine when the condition will emerge, how severe the course of illness will be, or whether treatment will be effective.

A detailed discussion of risks, benefits, and alternatives with attention to personal values is the core of informed consent. Genetic information is statistical and *probabilistic*. Risks are expressed as statistical probabilities and as such are extremely abstract concepts that are difficult to interpret and explain. Studies suggest that it is problematic to adequately describe the risks and benefits of genetic research or interventions to healthy persons or to those with medical illnesses. For persons with cognitive deficits, the meaning of genetic information may present more challenges.

Currently, no genetic interventions are available that can prevent, correct, or reverse the course of serious mental illnesses once they manifest. Researchers, patients, and clinicians must carefully weigh the psychological harm that may come from the knowledge of genetic status, given the absence of curative treatments and the uncertain benefits of early detection and treatment. Nevertheless, in the future, a test result suggesting greater vulnerability to developing schizophrenia or bipolar disorder may enable individuals and families to take preventive action, such as close monitoring of symptoms, avoidance of substance abuse and extreme stress that may trigger onset of a disorder, or even prophylactic or ameliorative pharmacology at the first signs of illness.

In providing consent information, most medical treatments or studies involve physical risks that can be stated in concrete terms of expected pain and discomfort. Genetic testing involves nothing more invasive than a cotton swab scraped across a cheek or, at most, the drawing of a blood sample. The risks are not biological per se; instead, there are psychosocial dangers to family relationships, the ability to obtain or maintain employment and health insurance. Many individuals with serious mental illnesses have problems with attention, memory, and processing that impair their comprehension of this kind of abstract and complicated information.

Information about genetic testing and genetic interventions also presents a challenge to affective dimensions of decisional capacity in psychiatric patients confronted with choices regarding genetic testing. Genetics as a subject arouses powerful emotions: guilt, fear, anxiety, despair, confusion, self-doubt, anger, and shame.

These feelings are amplified in conditions such as schizophrenia, bipolar disorder, and substance abuse. Finally, the familial nature of genetic testing and treatment may negatively affect the capacity for voluntarism. The entire topic of genetics may accentuate dysfunctional family dynamics. Families desperate for a cure may pressure patients to participate in genetic research that offers no real hope of intervention, while they may also prevent the patient from enrolling in genetic studies because of their own fear or guilt about what may be revealed.

■ CONFIDENTIALITY

Genetic data is *familial* data. Most contemporary psychiatric genetic research depends on pedigrees and often blood or tissue samples from family members of the person enrolled in genetic testing or treatment—the proband. Diagnosing an individual with bipolar disorder reveals information about the presence or susceptibility of the index condition and often of related psychiatric disorders in parents, siblings, children, and even those who have died or are yet to be born. Hence, the disclosure of genetic information can have an impact—for good and ill—at three levels: the individual, the family, and the community. Learning the results of genetic tests can cause great benefit or harm, depending upon the individuals' personality, the larger context, and the immediate circumstances. Some families will feel relief and a sense of control from being able to warn other family members and to make informed marital and reductive decisions. Other individuals may feel depressed, angry, and hopeless when they learn of a susceptibility to mental illness. They may blame their parents, God, or themselves and may feel that there is no sense in marrying, finishing their education, developing a career, or having children. Studies of genetic testing for Huntington's disease indicate that a minority of people become suicidal or refuse to be tested for fear of not being able to handle the results. Guilt, shame, withdrawal, and rage can all disrupt family relationships, as members will differ on whether or not they wished to know their genetic propensity to mental illness. Conversely, families who have negative tests may assume that they have little or no risk of mental illness and may ignore warning signs of decompensation and not seek treatment.

One of the most difficult confidentiality concerns in psychiatric genetics is whether investigators or clinicians should or must disclose the results of genetic testing to family members who are at risk of developing a serious mental illness. As part of the initial informed consent procedure in genetic research, the proband usually gives the investigators permission to contact his or her relatives to explain the study and to offer them participation. Researchers endeavor to protect the privacy and confidentially of all family members by revealing only the absolute minimum of information necessary to pursue the scientific goals of the study (Bonvicini 1998). What if family members who are at risk refuse contact with either the proband or the researchers? There is growing ethical and legal opinion that there is an obligation to contact relatives deemed to be at risk, even when the proband who serves as the research study participant refuses to provide consent for such contact (Deftos 1998). The case law on this point derives from *Tarasoff* and the duty to warn an identifiable victim and to take reasonable measures to protect them from harm. This evolving duty is highly controversial, as it contradicts traditional medical ethics precepts to respect the confidentiality and act in the best interests of the individual patient. Given that genetic data is perforce family data, the family may come to be seen ethically and treated clinically as a "unit" in psychiatric genetic work, equivalent to the individual patient in other forms of care. The therapeutic alliance will ironically become even more important in the age of genetic psychiatry, as clinicians struggle to balance the needs and wishes of patients and family members.

■ CONSIDERATIONS OF JUSTICE

Too often, when genetic information is revealed at the social and community level, the unfortunate result is stigma and discrimination. Because both the mentally ill and persons with medical genetic disease have already been documented objects of prejudice and injustice, persons with positive genetic findings for mental illness confront a double discrimination and overlapping vulnerabilities. A recent court case from Hong Kong illustrates the enormous discriminative potential of psychiatric genetic information (Wong and Lieh-Mak 2001). Three young men had applied to serve in various branches of the protective forces (e.g., the fire and customs departments). They were refused employment on the basis of a family history of schizophrenia, which was held to be an indicator of increased potential for violence. None of the applicants were symptomatic or had ever been diagnosed with a mental illness or received genetic testing. It turned out even a family history could only be substantiated in two of the cases. After testimony by numerous psychiatric genetic experts, the court ruled in favor of the plaintiffs. The court ruled that it was unlawful for the civil service to discriminate in employment, for the sake of public safety, against people with a family history of mental illness. The court further ruled that an individualized assessment of specific risks, rather than the application of population-based lifetime risks, must be applied in determining fitness for work (Wong and Lieh-Mak 2001).

This case and reported examples of people with only a risk of inherited medical disorders who have lost their health insurance, employment, or other educational and occupational opportunities underscore the need to protect genetic information from unauthorized disclosure to third parties who might use it to exploit or harm the individuals and their families (Billings et al. 1992). Even false-positive results and incorrectly interpreted findings have led to persons being unable to obtain health insurance for their children or be promoted at work (Lapham et al. 1996). Studies with patients who have a high risk of developing breast cancer show that fears of discrimination and stigmatization dissuade patients from participating in research and from seeking diagnosis and treatment until the disease has progressed (Armstrong et al. 2000).

Perhaps the most significant consideration of justice is that genetic information is *existential* and thus has import for our understanding of who we are as human beings, of where we have come from, and of what our destiny may be. Individuals may have their self-image, view of their possibilities and origins dramatically and tragically altered and suffer social stigmatization because they have a genetic variant that has been associated with mental illness.

■ EMPIRICAL STUDIES ON ETHICAL ISSUES IN PSYCHIATRIC GENETICS

To date, there are only four major studies of ethical issues in psychiatric genetics in published literature: three dealing with bipolar disorder and one with schizophrenia. Schulz et al. (1982) used the Family Attitudes Questionnaire to measure attitudes and perceptions toward the etiology, familial risk, and socioeconomic burden of schizophrenia, as well as childbearing plans and the acceptability of genetic counseling, in members of 17 families, each with a child with schizophrenia. The results revealed a disparity between the attitudes of well family members and the attitudes of patients: 92% of parents, compared with only 25% of patients, identified schizophrenia as an extremely burdensome disorder. Twenty-nine percent of parents, compared with 66% of ill persons, reported that they would have children based on their knowledge and experience of schizophrenia in their family.

Smith et al. (1996) investigated attitudes toward bipolar disorder and genetic testing, including prenatal testing and possible pregnancy termination related to course and severity of illness. Members of a bipolar support group, medical students, and psychiatry residents were surveyed. Nearly half of participants in the total sample ($n=93$) reported that they would terminate pregnancy if the fetus were definitely to develop an unspecified form of bipolar disorder. Presumed severity of illness was also found to be a modifying factor. Support group members were the least likely to say that they would terminate a hypothetical pregnancy in the case of a positive prenatal test and were the most likely to desire childhood testing in the absence of preventive or treatment options.

Targum et al. (1981) used the Family Attitudes Questionnaire to study the perceptions of 19 bipolar manic-depressive patients and their well spouses about the etiology, familial risk, and long-term burden of bipolar illness, marriage, and childbearing. In this study, 53% of well spouses, compared with only 5% of patients, reported that they would not have had children if they had known more about bipolar illness. In general, the data showed that the bipolar patients, compared with their spouse, minimized the burden and denied the heritable/familial nature of affective illness.

Trippitelli et al. (1998) performed a pilot study to examine the knowledge and attitudes of individuals with bipolar disorder and their spouses ($N=90$) regarding treatment response rates for bipolar disorder, probability of inheritance, genetic testing, disclosure of genetic information, abortion, marriage, and childbearing. The majority of the patients and spouses said that they would use genetic tests for bipolar disorder if they were available. Most patients and spouses felt that the benefits of knowledge of carrying a bipolar gene outweighed the risks. Few respondents also would abort a fetus carrying a gene for bipolar disorder, nor would prior knowledge that they carried a bipolar gene have dissuaded most patients or spouses from marriage or childbearing.

■ GENETIC COUNSELING FOR PSYCHIATRIC DISORDERS

The findings of these studies indicate that despite the inherent psychosocial risks of genetic testing and interventions for mental illness, a substantial number of patients and family members will be interested in obtaining genetic services when they become clinically accessible. Competent and compassionate genetic counseling will be essential to maximize the therapeutic benefits of genetic research, testing, and therapy while minimizing the adverse consequences. Unfortunately, there is a projected shortage of trained genetic counselors who will be restricted to academic settings and to performing a consultative function (Holtzman 1993). It is clinical psychiatrists and neurologists, and possibly primary care clinicians, who will be charged with the task of counseling psychiatric patients and families about the promise and peril of genetics in the coming decades (Stancer and Wagener 1984).

Clinicians can take several steps to begin to develop the knowledge and skills needed for genetic counseling of psychiatric patients (Table 12–1). First, the decisional capacity and voluntarism of mentally ill persons to consent to genetic testing, research, and therapy must be prudently assessed, methodically respected, and patiently facilitated. Clinicians may need to have a series of discussions about genetic risks and benefits; utilize audiovisual materials, analogies, and problem-solving exercises to convey the valence of probabilities; and evaluate the need for a surrogate decision maker. Second, clinicians need to invite and enhance family involvement from the initial stages of discussion and in an ongoing fashion, both to safeguard the autonomy, privacy, and confidentiality of all parties and to allow the "family patient" to receive the best care possible. It will be crucial to clarify personal, familial, and social values relevant to the decisions to be made. Third, most practicing psychiatrists and neurologists will have received at most a rudimentary training in psychiatric genetics, and few psychologists, nurses, counselors, and social workers will have received even this level of preparation. Nevertheless, they can avail themselves of the burgeoning continuing medical education in genetics and the ethical, legal, religious, and social implications of genetic research offered through the Internet, conferences, books, and journals. Fifth, clinicians can identify experts in ethics, religion, culture, and/or genetics at local university hospitals or research centers or ethics committees whom they may consult on an informal and formal basis. Clinicians who follow these and other constructive suggestions will be well situated to apply the fruits of genetic research to the clinical care of patients with scientific rigor and ethical responsibility.

TABLE 12–1.	**Means of increasing knowledge and skill in clinical psychiatric genetics**

Always take a detailed family history, which includes seeking collateral information if patients give permission.

Carefully assess and monitor the decisional capacity and voluntarism of patients seeking genetic testing.

Use analogy, repeated discussions, and audiovisual materials to illustrate risk and probability.

Work to involve the family, to clarify family and relevant personal, cultural, and social values, and to obtain consent for the sharing of results.

Identify and obtain appropriate consultation.

Participate in continuing education on psychiatric genetics.

Case Scenarios

A 28-year-old construction worker whose mother was institutionalized for schizophrenia wants to enroll in a genetic study of the condition to decide whether he should ever get married or have children.

A 46-year-old mother of two grown children whose own mother died of early-onset Alzheimer's requests genetic testing for the disease. When discussing the possibility of a positive test with the counselor, she states that she would kill herself before becoming seriously "demented."

A 25-year-old journalist mentions to her physician that there is a family history of bipolar disorder. A month later, her insurance is canceled, stating she did not reveal a preexisting condition when disclosing her prior history to the company.

A 35-year-old man is a nurse manager at a community hospital. He has never had a drinking problem, but his father had severe and unremitting alcohol addiction until his death. The son chooses to enroll in a genetic study of alcoholism because he is concerned about his own teenage children. He later informs the physician at the occupational health clinic of his involvement in the protocol. Shortly thereafter, he is placed on "probation for alcoholism," since his workplace medical record states that he was in an "alcoholism study."

Case Scenarios *(continued)*

A 27-year-old computer engineer is offered a job with a high-security technology firm. He had briefly been treated for depression as a graduate student and had a grandmother who committed suicide. When the company physician reviews his mental health history, the previous offer of employment is withdrawn.

■ REFERENCES

Armstrong K, Calzone K, Stopfer J, et al: Factors associated with decisions about clinical BRCA1/2 testing. Cancer Epidemiol Biomarkers Prev 9:1251–1254, 2000

Billings PR, Kohn MA, de Cuevas M, et al: Discrimination as a consequence of genetic testing. Am J Hum Genet 50:476–482, 1992

Bonvicini KA: The art of recruitment: the foundation of family and linkage studies of psychiatric illness. Fam Process 37:153–165, 1998

Deftos LJ: The evolving duty to disclose the presence of genetic disease to relatives. Acad Med 73:962–968, 1998

Holtzman NA: Primary care physicians as providers of frontline genetic services. Fetal Diagn Ther 8 (suppl 1):213–219, 1993

Lapham EV, Kozma C, Weiss JO: Genetic discrimination: perspectives of consumers. Science 274:621–624, 1996

National Institute of Mental Health Genetics Workgroup: Genetics and Mental Disorders. Bethesda, MD, National Institute of Mental Health, 1997

Schulz PM, Schulz SC, Dibble E, et al: Patient and family attitudes about schizophrenia: implications for genetic counseling. Schizophr Bull 8: 504–513, 1982

Smith LB, Sapers B, Reus VI, et al: Attitudes towards bipolar disorder and predictive genetic testing among patients and providers. J Med Genet 33:544–549, 1996

Stancer HC, Wagener DK: Genetic counselling: its need in psychiatry and the directions it gives for future research. Can J Psychiatry 29:289–294, 1984

Targum SD, Dibble ED, Davenport YB, et al: The Family Attitudes Questionnaire. Patients' and spouses' views of bipolar illness. Arch Gen Psychiatry 38:562–568, 1981

Trippitelli CL, Jamison KR, Folstein MF, et al: Pilot study on patients' and spouses' attitudes toward potential genetic testing for bipolar disorder. Am J Psychiatry 155:899–904, 1998

Wong JG, Lieh-Mak F: Genetic discrimination and mental illness: a case report. J Med Ethics 27:393–397, 2001

ETHICAL ISSUES IN MANAGED AND EVOLVING SYSTEMS OF CARE

Systems of health care in this country are rapidly evolving, and perceptions of what constitutes ethically sound care within these systems are changing as well. Beyond ethics principles governing the care of individual patients, there is a new emphasis on principles of ethics that relate to resource distribution and social justice issues across patient populations. Meeting the needs of individual patients while wisely shepherding scarce resources has been identified as a component of the profession of medicine's "social contract" (McCurdy et al. 1997; "Medical Professionalism in the New Millennium" 2002).

Balancing the health care needs of populations with the health care needs of individuals, however, has created real and often unforeseen ethical binds for clinicians in both the private and the public sectors. Managed care organizations in particular have been identified as disrupting the clinician–patient relationship, which traditionally has been based on the patient's ability to choose a clinician, on clinician competence, on communication and compassion in the clinical relationship, on continuity of care, and on the absence of conflicts of interest (Hall 1997). Moreover, as resource priorities have been made within society and within new systems of care, stigma and poor recognition of the importance of mental illness have acted together to diminish resources for people with psychiatric and comorbid disease. Patients with mental illness—

individuals who have always posed special challenges in the provision of clinical services—are now encountering heightened obstacles to adequate treatment in these new systems of care. In this chapter we define specific ethical principles and values that should guide the development of mental health service systems, outline ethically important features of mental health services, and discuss strategies for addressing ethical conflicts in evolving systems of care.

■ ETHICAL PRINCIPLES IN MANAGED AND EVOLVING SYSTEMS OF CARE

There are several critically important ethics principles that should guide the development and implementation of mental health services (Table 13–1). *Respect for persons* is the principle that ensures that the dignity and the basic rights of individual patients will be recognized and upheld in interactions and procedures within a system of care. Closely related to this concept is the notion of *autonomy*—supporting the ability of the individual patient to make informed, independent decisions regarding his or her own physical body and emotional self. The professional duty to respect the individual's right to self-governance does not mean that clinicians must provide everything that patients desire or request. Nevertheless, in some health care settings, patient autonomy may not be sufficiently supported because patients receive marked pressure to accept certain kinds of treatments that are convenient or less expensive (e.g., medication) rather than treatments that are more in keeping with the patient's personal beliefs and values (e.g., psychotherapy or combined psychosocial and biological interventions).

Integrity refers to the consistent fulfillment by the clinician, both in word and in behavior, of the ideals of the profession of medicine. This means, for example, that the patient's well-being and best interests should be the clinician's primary concern (i.e., *beneficence*). Moreover, with rare exceptions as noted below, the system should support the clinician's ability to help each patient according to current standards of care, faithfully seeking to ameliorate and al-

TABLE 13–1. Ethical principles in systems of care

Ethical principle	Application to systems of care
Respect for persons: ensures that the dignity and rights of the individual are recognized and upheld	In its interactions and procedures, the system should recognize the dignity and uphold the rights of the patient
Autonomy: supports the ability of the individual to make informed, independent decisions about his or her body and self	The system should sufficiently support patient autonomy so that patients are not pressured to accept treatments contrary to their values because of expense or expedience. This does not mean that clinicians must provide what patients desire or request
Integrity: consistent adherence to the ideals of the medical profession	The system should support the principle that the patient's best interests are the clinician's primary goal
Beneficence: the patient's well-being is the physician's central concern	The system should support the clinician's ability to • Adhere to high standards of care • Alleviate suffering • Provide cure where possible
Fidelity: faithfulness to the ideals of medicine and the good of the patient	Clinicians need to be wary of conflicts of interest, such as where the system proffers • Economic incentives to provide minimal services or substandard treatment • Contracts specifying that reimbursement is contingent upon withholding of care

TABLE 13–1. Ethical principles in systems of care *(continued)*

Ethical principle	Application to systems of care
Veracity: truthfulness in the physician–patient relationship	Clinicians need to be wary of system contracts that threaten honesty (e.g., nondisclosure clauses that require physicians not to inform patients of superior treatment available outside the system)
Confidentiality: the positive duty to protect personal information in the absence of patient consent or legal exceptions	The issues are highly complex and overlapping in managed care systems, and employers or insurers may be informed of personal health information
Fairness: the ideal of social justice in which goods, harms, and burdens are equitably distributed	The enormous income of for-profit systems may be obtained at the cost of providing substandard care, especially to ill individuals without alternatives

leviate suffering and to provide curative treatments wherever possible (i.e., *fidelity*). Financial conflicts of interest, such as economic incentives to clinicians for providing minimal services and substandard treatment, represent significant threats to the integrity and fidelity of clinicians. Clinicians should be very wary of managed care organizations that proffer contracts that contain provisions specifying, for example, that the reimbursement plan is contingent upon withholding care (e.g., limiting tests ordered or numbers or kinds of prescriptions written).

Veracity, or truthfulness, is a fundamental value within medicine, and it is also threatened by practices within some systems of care. For instance, contracts that include nondisclosure clauses requiring that clinicians not inform patients of standard or superior treatments that are available outside of their system are in violation of this professional duty to deal with patients honestly. *Confidentiality* is the positive duty to protect the personal information of patients and not to disclose this information in the absence either of clear permission from the patient or of regulatory or legal mandates (e.g., compulsory reporting of child abuse or of serious infectious disease). In many systems of care related to employment settings, for example, confidentiality issues become highly complex as supervisors are informed of the personal health information of employees routinely, as is now emerging in many workplaces in which genetic testing is conducted.

Finally, *fairness* in resource allocation is the ethics principle that poses the greatest challenge in many of the newly emerging health care systems. Fairness derives from the ideal of social justice, which states that goods, harms, and burdens of society should be shared by individuals who exist within different segments of society in an equitable, if not equal, manner. Systems of health care are often assessed in relation to the issue of fairness. For example, universal health insurance is one policy initiative that has been advanced on the basis of a social justice rationale. The very striking financial gains attained by some for-profit managed care systems that provide substandard clinical care have been criticized on the grounds that they are fundamentally unfair to the ill individuals within their systems, who may not have other viable alternatives for care.

■ EVOLVING SYSTEMS OF CARE FOR MENTAL ILLNESS

To be clinically effective and ethically sound, health services optimally will be adapted to address the specific nature and core attributes of the health issues of the people served. First, ideally, mental health services will be structured to respond to the high prevalence of mental disorders and the frequency of comorbidity with medical and substance-related disorders. Specifically, the Epidemiologic Catchment Area (ECA) survey assessed the 1-year incidence of mental disorders among adults ages 18 years and older as 12.3% (Regier et al. 1993). The National Comorbidity Study (NCS) of 8,000 adults ages 15–54 years revealed a 1-year incidence rate of mental disorders of 30% and a lifetime prevalence of 48% (Kessler et al. 1994). In both the ECA survey and the NCS, the most common disorders overall were alcohol abuse or dependence, phobias (i.e., an anxiety disorder), and major depression.

Symptoms of mental illness are highly prominent in general clinic settings, as has been shown in studies by Leon et al., Regier et al., Spitzer et al., and Johnson et al., who found that between 30% and 45% of primary care patients had diagnosable mental disorders (Johnson et al. 1995; Olfson et al. 1997; Spitzer et al. 1995). More than 50% of patients with any mental illness are treated exclusively within a primary care setting (Kamerow 1986). In addition, it is estimated that 10%–25% of patients in primary care settings have alcohol or other substance abuse problems (Andreasen and Black 2001). Interestingly, as mental health treatment access has decreased over the past decade, costs have shifted to the medical health care "side" of many systems of care. Tanielian et al. (1997), for instance, found that the number of general hospital discharges with a documented primary mental disorder rose from 1.41 million to 1.67 million between 1988 and 1993. This increase of 18.3% is dramatically higher than the rise of discharges with a primary diagnosis of a general medical disorder, 0.1%, during the same time period.

On the basis of these studies and other epidemiological data, it is estimated that at least 15 million Americans will suffer from a significant mental disorder at one time or another in their lives and that between 1.7 and 4 million Americans are seriously mentally ill at a given time. About 900,000 of these individuals reside in institutional or community settings, and a large proportion are homeless.

Second, beyond the simple recognition of the burden of need for mental health care, evolving systems ideally will be responsive to the psychosocial and societal impact of mental illness. It is well documented that individuals with mental illness have diminished overall quality of life and, by definition, some compromise in interpersonal and social roles (Penn and Martin 1998). Moreover, the symptoms of some mental illnesses, such as amotivation, apathy, mistrust, impaired insight, and poor relatedness, may serve as barriers to pursuit of care. This is especially true in systems in which patients must navigate a series of gatekeeping steps before being seen by a mental health specialist. Beyond the level of individual suffering, the societal effects of mental illness are substantial. The Surgeon General's report estimated that mental disorders collectively account for more than 15% of the overall burden of disease in the United States. This burden is greater than the burden from all other causes and slightly more than the burden associated with all forms of cancer (U.S. Department of Health and Human Services 1999). The World Health Organization's (WHO's) Global Burden of Disease study found that mental illness, including suicide, ranks second in the burden of disease in industrialized nations. The WHO study discovered that research that examined only deaths vastly underestimated the negative impact of mental illness on quality of life. The WHO therefore used a method of comparing disease burden known as disability-adjusted life years (DALYs). DALYs assign a value to premature death and to severity and length of disability. When DALYs were used, major depression ranked second only to ischemic heart disease in magnitude of disease burden. Schizophrenia, bipolar disorder, obsessive-compulsive disorder, panic disorder, and posttraumatic stress disorder also contributed significantly to the burden represented by mental illness (Murray and Lopez 1996). These disturbing data highlight the immediacy and significance of mental health as a public health problem and strongly argue for increases in the resources allocated for diagnosis and treatment of mental illness.

Finally, ethically sound systems of mental health services will be adapted to the need for scientific study and educational training related to these poorly understood, devastating disorders. Academic medical centers, which traditionally have provided care for large segments of the chronically mentally ill population in this country, for instance, are now struggling to survive financially. The broad educational missions of most departments of psychiatry in this country, however, have been limited over the past several years as the prominence of for-profit managed care organizations has emerged. These 126, primarily urban, health care centers are estimated to provide 50% of the uncompensated care in the United States. Many of these academic medical centers exist in states with managed Medicaid programs, making adequate funding for community based services even more elusive (Stout 1998). Clinical service now drives most faculty career paths as research funds have decreased significantly; for example, whereas in the 1960s, 40% of a medical school's revenues derived from research, in 1990, that proportion had diminished to 17% (Riba and Tasman 1993). With the financial restructuring of these academic departments, research and training programs have been severely and negatively affected, a situation that bodes poorly for future care of mentally ill individuals in this country (Meyer et al. 1998).

■ RESOLVING CONFLICTS BETWEEN THE NEEDS OF INDIVIDUALS AND POPULATIONS

Within the currently evolving systems of care in our society, legitimate ethical conflicts may arise between the clinical needs of the individual patient and the shared clinical resource needs of a larger set of individuals. In such situations, key principles such as respect for persons, truth telling, fairness, and confidentiality should not be compromised. The physician's commitment is to improve quality of care and access to care, to foster just distribution of finite resources, and to maintain trust by managing conflicts of interest. Additional efforts to enhance the process of clinical care and to clarify the values governing resource-rationing decisions are essential to ethically sound care in these systems, however. For instance, when an individual patient is not provided with an optimal or even a standard treatment for a particular illness, the reasons for this decision must be made explicit and clarified on both individual and community levels.

Some managed care organizations have also been criticized for their practices, which interfere with informed consent in such "rationing" situations. For example, the quality of communication and information exchange between clinician and patient may be compromised by time constraints, inaccessibility of a consistent care provider, perceived "double agentry," and "gag rules." On a broader level, ideally, there will be a community assent process for any large resource decisions affecting individual patient care, and alternative avenues for care will be identified and publicized. One example of this might be the decision, in a region with high levels of poverty and a capitated Medicaid system, to limit the availability of doctoral-level mental health specialists for adults but to retain these services for children. To be faithful to the aim of social justice, however, people with mental illness must be included and their viewpoints adequately represented in the process of this decision— a very rare occurrence in nearly all systems in which allocation and rationing choices are made.

In light of these ethical conflicts primarily related to resource distribution, Hall (1997) proposed several prerequisites for an optimal health delivery system. These prerequisites aim to prevent and resolve problems that emerge when individuals are competing for resources within the managed system. Hall indicated that the system must be patient responsive, provide adequate and compassionate care, encourage physician excellence, be accessible, reduce bureaucracy to a minimum, provide humane treatment based on scientific merit, and be accountable to the patient. Some authors have further suggested that optimal and ethical systems will place significant emphasis on prevention and early illness interventions, which are relatively cost-effective at the population level and yet greatly benefit individual patients (Haas 1997). Though scarce, managed care systems that support scientific inquiry are increasingly recognized as important ethically in light of the crippling impact of managed care systems upon scientific activities at academic medical centers in this country (Billi et al. 1995; Kralewski et al. 1995; Mechanic and Dobson 1996).

Similarly, Sabin (1996) proposed four ethical premises of managed mental health care specifically in resolving resource conflicts:

1. Ethical clinicians should dedicate themselves to caring for their patients in a relationship of fidelity and at the same time act as stewards of society's resources.
2. Ethical clinicians should recommend the least costly treatment alternative unless they have substantial evidence that a more costly intervention is likely to yield a superior outcome.
3. In their stewardship role, ethical clinicians need to advocate for justice in the health care system, just as in their clinical role they need to advocate for the welfare of their patients.
4. Ethical clinicians insist that potentially beneficial interventions should be withheld only on the basis of explicit standards that have been established with the participation of the affected populations and that are acknowledged by the individual patient.

Sabin further suggested that these ethical premises place special responsibilities on clinicians and the public to insist that managed health systems truly improve the effectiveness of care (i.e., improve outcomes in relation to resources spent). Moreover, he stated that clinicians and the public must insist that a genuine informed consent process occur nationally, regionally, in communities, and with patients. Finally, clinicians and the public must "demand that all

Americans have access to an adequate standard of health care." Failure to pursue these steps will ultimately lead to unethical conduct by clinicians, as they will have participated in a system of care that is not beneficent, honest, or just (Sabin 1996).

In sum, the newly emerging managed systems of mental health care in this country are not inherently unethical, but they do pose special ethical problems as the needs of individuals come into conflict with the needs of populations. Indeed, many believe that the prudent shepherding of health care resources congruent with ethical principles such as respect for persons, autonomy, beneficence, and social justice is itself a new moral imperative in our society. Nevertheless, focused attention on practices, policies, and conflict-resolution strategies is essential to ethically sound care for individuals with mental illness within evolving systems of care.

Case Scenarios

A patient is no longer suicidal but requires several more days to stabilize in the hospital after a mixed bipolar episode. The health maintenance organization refuses to pay for a longer stay. The psychiatrist writes in the notes, "Patient continues to be at high risk of suicide."

Clinicians at an academic medical center are told that patients with newly diagnosed depression can only be treated with a single medication unless they fail a trial or have severe side effects from the first-line medication on the formulary, because offering alternative medications is too expensive.

A child psychiatrist must decide whether to send an 8-year-old boy with psychotic symptoms out of state, because there are no beds in his region. The parents cannot afford to accompany the child.

A partial hospital program is told by the administration that it will be closed if it cannot demonstrate improved outcomes and shortened stays for the dually diagnosed patients in its program.

An insurance company denies a claim for psychotherapy from a psychiatrist treating a woman for severe social phobia, but tells the patient it will pay for six sessions with a social worker.

■ REFERENCES

Andreasen NC, Black DW: Introductory Textbook of Psychiatry. Washington DC, American Psychiatric Press, 2001

Billi JE, Wise CG, Bills EA, et al: Potential effects of managed care on specialty practice at a university medical center [see comments]. N Engl J Med 333:979–983, 1995

Haas BK: The effect of managed care on breast cancer detection, treatment, and research. Nurs Outlook 45:167–172, 1997

Hall RC: Ethical and legal implications of managed care. Gen Hosp Psychiatry 19:200–208, 1997

Johnson JG, Spitzer RL, Williams JB, et al: Psychiatric comorbidity, health status, and functional impairment associated with alcohol abuse and dependence in primary care patients: findings of the PRIME MD-1000 study. J Consult Clin Psychol 63:133–140, 1995

Kamerow DB: Research on mental disorders in primary care settings: rationale, topics, and support. Fam Pract Res J 6:5–11, 1986

Kessler RC, McGonagle KA, Zhao S, et al: Lifetime and 12-month prevalence of DSM-III-R psychiatric disorders in the United States. Results from the National Comorbidity Survey. Arch Gen Psychiatry 51:8–19, 1994

Kralewski JE, Hart G, Perlmutter C, et al: Can academic medical centers compete in a managed care system? Acad Med 70:867–872, 1995

McCurdy L, Goode LD, Inui TS, et al: Fulfilling the social contract between medical schools and the public. Acad Med 72:1063–1070, 1997

Mechanic RE, Dobson A: The impact of managed care on clinical research: a preliminary investigation. Health Aff (Millwood) 15:72–89, 1996

Medical professionalism in the new millennium: a physician charter. ABIM Foundation, ACP-ASIM Foundation, European Federation of Internal Medicine. Ann Intern Med 136:243–246, 2002

Meyer M, Genel M, Altman RD, et al: Clinical research: assessing the future in a changing environment; summary report of conference sponsored by the American Medical Association Council on Scientific Affairs, Washington, DC, March 1996. Am J Med 104:264–271, 1998

Murray JL, Lopez AD (eds): The Global Burden of Disease. A Comprehensive Assessment of Mortality and Disability From Diseases, Injuries, and Risk Factors in 1990 and Projected to 2020. Cambridge, MA, Harvard School of Public Health, 1996

Olfson M, Fireman B, Weissman MM, et al: Mental disorders and disability among patients in a primary care group practice. Am J Psychiatry 154:1734–1740, 1997

Penn DL, Martin J: The stigma of severe mental illness: some potential solutions for a recalcitrant problem. Psychiatr Q 69:235–247, 1998

Regier DA, Narrow WE, Rae DS, et al: The de facto US mental and addictive disorders service system. Epidemiologic Catchment Area prospective 1-year prevalence rates of disorders and services. Arch Gen Psychiatry 50:85–94, 1993

Riba M, Tasman A: Investor-owned psychiatric hospitals and universities: can their marriage succeed? Hosp Community Psychiatry 44:547–550, 1993

Sabin J: Is managed care ethical? in Controversies in Managed Mental Health Care. Edited by Lazarus A. Washington, DC, American Psychiatric Press, 1996, pp 115–128

Spitzer RL, Kroenke K, Linzer M, et al: Health-related quality of life in primary care patients with mental disorders. Results from the PRIME-MD 1000 Study. JAMA 274:1511–1517, 1995

Stout M: Impact of Medicaid managed mental health care on delivery of services in a rural state: an AMI perspective. Psychiatr Serv 49:961–963, 1998

Tanielian TL, Pincus HA, Olfson M, et al: General hospital discharges of patients with mental and physical disorders. Psychiatr Serv 48:311, 1997

U.S. Department of Health and Human Services: Mental Health: A Report of the Surgeon General. Rockville, MD, U.S. Department of Health and Human Services, 1999

14

ETHICAL ISSUES IN CLINICIAN HEALTH

With Merry N. Miller, M.D.

Caregivers in the arena of mental health face enormous personal burdens as part of a profession that cannot be practiced impersonally. It is estimated that a psychotherapist has 10 productive years before burnout and disillusionment from working intensively with the psychological suffering of others overtakes the idealism that motivated most people to enter a helping profession in the first place (Grosch and Olsen 1994) (Table 14–1). Mental health care professionals suffer from stress and stress-related disorders; substance abuse; depression, sometimes ending in suicide; personal and family problems, often leading to divorce—at rates that often exceed those among the population at large. Medical students and residents become exhausted; they have little time to establish patterns of preventive health; they are vulnerable to addiction, mental illness, and relationship problems; and they may fear academic repercussions if they acknowledge being ill or seeking personal health care (Roberts et al. 2001). Physicians are more than twice as likely as the general population to commit suicide ("Physician Suicide" 1987; Sargent 1987). Each year, it would take the equivalent of one or two average-sized graduating classes of medical students to replace the number of physicians who kill themselves.

This is obviously a tragedy of enormous personal, professional, and societal dimensions. From the standpoint of ethics, we

TABLE 14–1. Symptoms of burnout

Physical	Behavioral	Psychological	Spiritual	Clinical
Fatigue	Loss of enthusiasm	Depression	Loss of faith	Cynicism towards clients
Physical depletion	Coming late to work	Emptiness	Loss of meaning	Daydreaming during sessions
Irritability	Accomplishing little despite long hours	Negative self-concept	Loss of purpose	Hostility toward clients
Headaches	Quickness to frustration and anger	Pessimism	Feelings of alienation	Boredom toward clients
Gastrointestinal disturbances	Becoming increasingly rigid	Guilt	Feelings of estrangement	Quickness to diagnose
Back pain	Difficulty making decisions	Self-blame for not accomplishing more	Changes in religious beliefs	Blaming clients
Weight change	Closing out new input	Feelings of omnipotence	Changes in religious affiliation	
Change in sleep pattern	Increased dependence on/withdrawal from colleagues			
	Irritation with co-workers			

Source. Modified from Grosch WN, Olsen DC: *When Helping Starts to Hurt: A New Look at Burnout Among Psychotherapists.* New York, WW Norton, 1994. Copyright 1994, WW Norton. Used with permission.

must consider a number of issues: 1) the ethical "obligation" to care for oneself—the ethical imperative as society's caretakers to keep healthy, both physically and emotionally; 2) ethical dilemmas in caring for professional colleagues and their families; 3) professional obligations to intervene when aware of an impaired professional and personal obligations to help a distressed colleague; and 4) the ethics of medicine's culture, which has traditionally rewarded self-denial and workaholism at the expense of healthy relationships and self-care.

The personal toll on clinicians from a career in one of the helping professions can be extreme. The overall physician suicide rate has been estimated to be more than twice that of the general population, and among female physicians the risk is especially high, with suicide rates that are four times higher than those for females in the general population (Council on Scientific Affairs 1987). The prevalence of depression and substance abuse among physicians appears to be similar to that in the general population, with increased rates among trainees (Miller and McGowen 2000). Divorce rates among physicians have been reported to be 10% to 20% higher than those in the general population (Sotile and Sotile 1996).

Despite the clear presence of serious mental health problems among professionals, many who need treatment do not get it. Denial is common, and the stigma many associate with psychiatric illness prevents many even within the field from getting help. In a study of 1,027 medical students at nine medical schools, Roberts et al. (2000, 2001) showed that although most medical students (90%) needed or wanted personal health care, nearly half had difficulty with access to care despite having insurance. A majority (57%) did not seek care at times, in part because of demands in the training situation, such as having no time to obtain care and worries about confidentiality. Students acknowledged substantial fear of reprisal for having or seeking care for stigmatizing illnesses. Finally, this study revealed that when presented with scenarios depicting students with evidence of very serious illness (e.g., suicidal depression, severe substance dependence, uncontrolled diabetes), roughly one-third of students opted to protect the student/colleague's confidentiality rather than intervene to help him get care or to report him to the dean's office. In this study, the pattern of self-diagnosis and curbside consultation for medical treatment was documented to occur early in the clinical training years. The repercussions of these mental health problems among clinicians are widespread and include potential effects on patient care in addition to the obvious effects on individual clinicians and their families.

Responding to the mental health problems of professional colleagues brings with it a number of ethical dilemmas and personal challenges. First, recognition that a colleague may be in need of help raises questions about the level of intervention that is appropriate. It is easy for colleagues to collude with the "impaired" clinician in terms of denial and minimization. Overidentification may also result in an exaggerated concern about the impact of treatment on the impaired clinician's career. Aggressive interventions such as involuntary hospitalization for the seriously suicidal colleague may be less likely due to a perceived conflict between the ethical obligation to protect the colleague's career and reputation versus the duty to protect the colleague's safety. Confidentiality issues can also become problematic in such situations. It is accepted that the need for safety takes precedence over confidentiality concerns, but professionals may hesitate to apply this rule when the patient is also a professional colleague. Limit setting can also be more difficult when treating professional colleagues. The boundaries that are normally maintained between physician and patient may be easily blurred when the patient is a professional colleague. Such boundary crossings may lead to increased strain on the caregiver and sometimes may result in inappropriate behaviors.

■ THE WOUNDED HEALER

The very qualities that attract people to the helping professions and make them good at what they do also make them vulnerable to the demands of the work. Empathy, sympathy, intuition, thoroughness, a strong work ethic, perfectionism, and the ability to absorb, tolerate and understand feelings are all qualities that are valuable in the helping professions. The willingness to take on the problems of others is seen as a mark of virtue. Yet there must be limits; the ability to help is not without bounds. One important boundary is the clinician's need to care for him- or herself.

Grosch and Olsen (1994), in their excellent review of burnout, *When Helping Starts to Hurt,* offered a useful perspective on the problems psychotherapists and other helping professionals face. They reviewed self psychology, particularly the work of Heinz Kohut, in delineating how a stable sense of self develops, how that self may be useful in doing the work of psychotherapy, and how it may be vulnerable to the demands of helping others (Kohut 1981, 1984). There are limits, and these limits between self and other are properly understood as boundaries. They are the boundaries that become so important in the therapeutic relationship, the boundaries between self and other, not just in a physical sense, but also in terms of maintaining the emotional ability to accurately reflect or mirror the other and to distinguish wants and desires.

The myth of Narcissus is relevant not just because he lent his name to this condition of vulnerability, narcissistic vulnerability. Narcissus has become the mythic figure of psychotherapy not because he fell in love with his image reflected in the pond, but because he needed the reassurance of a reflection of himself, just as people need an accurate reflection of themselves when they enter psychotherapy.

Reciprocally, therapists need that same mirroring and often seek and find it in their work. They may be appreciated for what they do—for their ability to help people to understand their own lives. However, equally likely, they may be frustrated by their inability to make things right for patients or clients, whose expectations of them may know no realistic bounds. This is the delicate work of therapy. Just as the ideal mother must ultimately frustrate the child she loves (because the child must ultimately face the outside world), so must the work of therapy ultimately frustrate the patient's wishes to be perfectly mirrored. Winnicott reminded us that what was needed was "good-enough mothering" or parenting. The perfect is the enemy of the good. Therapists can be vulnerable to a personal need for appreciation, to feelings of failure in cases where an attempt to rescue or to set things right was unsuccessful, to the desire to be a better parent themselves, or to grandiose or exaggerated self-expectations (Winnicott 1964). Conversely, there can be great rewards in therapy (as in parenting) by being empathic enough to understand and help the patient understand the limitations of the therapy and of living life.

■ THE PATH TO WELLNESS

Perfectionistic expectations probably represent the greatest resistance to treatment in patients and among professionals. For those conditioned to appear self-reliant, getting help seems an admission of weakness. Affects of shame and thoughts of doubt accompany the recognition of the need for help, the first steps toward treatment, and at least the early phases of the process of psychotherapy.

Mental health begins and ends with self-awareness. Indeed, an important aspect of the talking cure has always been the imperative to examine one's own life. Psychoanalysis continually holds before us the possibility that there are aspects of ourselves that remain out of awareness—unconscious (Table 14–2).

TABLE 14–2. **The path to wellness**

Self-awareness
Self-help
Supervision or consultation
Support groups
Psychotherapy
Family-of-origin work
Inpatient treatment
Self-awareness

■ THE VIP SYNDROME

Even when clinicians do seek help, they are often treated differently from other patients. Colleagues may be treated as "very important persons" (VIPs) and may actually receive less-than-optimal care because exceptions are made for them, their denials accepted, confrontations are avoided. They may receive less aggressive treatment than is really needed, possibly because of overidentification with the patient on the part of the treating physician (Stoudemire and Rhoads 1983). Being a VIP may also increase a clinician's sense of shame and resistance to treatment. Those who see themselves and who are seen by others as "important" and strong may have more difficulty admitting their own problems and identifying themselves as in need of help. They also may be more likely to try to control and direct the treatment.

Clearly, clinicians are VIPs, but so are all patients. VIPs should receive the same excellent care that anyone else would receive. Treating clinicians may recognize that the clinicians they treat are special to them, but as an ethical principle, providers should strive to give everyone the care they need. This nondiscriminatory principle is useful as a reminder of the responsibility to serve egalitarian ends in treating the difficult patient, the indigent patient, or other unique persons. It can also serve as a reminder not to provide inferior care to patients just because they are either very similar to or very different from ourselves.

■ THE IMPAIRED PROFESSIONAL

Impairment in the context of professional ethics is defined as the inability to provide clinical care with reasonable skill and safety to patients by reason of physical or mental illness or substance dependence. Awareness of impairment and of the ethical and legal duties associated with colleague impairment are also important ethics skills for clinicians. Impairment is a spectrum disorder ranging from mild forms to more severe. Worry and preoccupation with day-to-day problems may prevent a clinician from being optimally empathic and go largely unnoticed. Persistent inattentiveness may be noticed by supervisors if the clinician is in training. The supervisor may inquire as to what is interfering with the ability to attend to the patient (or client) and encourage therapy if appropriate. Self-scrutiny thus becomes one of the objectives of the training experience. More severe impediments to effective practice include addictions and mental illness.

In the past, addictions and mental illness were seen as moral shortcomings and were dealt with accordingly through punitive measures. We may identify such attitudes with remote periods of history, but in fact they persist today. A therapeutic approach to impaired professionals is only gradually overcoming the older, more pejorative attitudes. Most states have now passed impaired-professional legislation, based on the model impaired-physician statute developed by the American Medical Association Council on Mental Health in the early 1970s. These legislative mandates provide a therapeutic alternative to loss of licensure for impaired professionals. Typically, an impaired professional voluntarily surrenders her or his license and agrees to enter a treatment program. Upon successful completion of the treatment, the license is restored with whatever monitoring may be deemed necessary.

The important thing to stress when dealing with impaired professionals is that improvement is possible, even dramatic improvement; that improvement involves talking about feelings and coming to accept and tolerate unpleasant feelings (especially shame and guilt); and that getting better is a social phenomenon. One cannot practice alone and one cannot get better without the help of other human beings.

Clinician health rests on this important principle. We may reply to the Biblical admonition, "Physician, heal thyself," with a modern caveat: "Heal thyself, but don't try to do it all by yourself."

■ CLINICIAN HEALTH AND TRAINING

The training process for clinicians is one that raises many ethical dilemmas. Training programs are known to be physically and emotionally stressful, often involving long working hours and even sleep deprivation. During medical school and residency, physicians learn to distance themselves from patients, to take on more and more work without complaint, and to compartmentalize their feelings. In addition, many practice settings reward long hours and self-neglect. Perfectionism and workaholic standards are pervasive in medicine and may play a role in the increased rates of distress seen among clinicians. Obsessionality, which is not the same thing as thoroughness, is seen as a virtue rather than what may be a defense against unpleasant emotions. Physicians essentially are taught to ignore their own needs if they want to be successful, and they may later have difficulty achieving balance in their lives.

The culture of medicine that has traditionally promoted an ideal of self-denial and workaholic standards is now being challenged. The Accreditation Council for Graduate Medical Education (2002) has proposed new regulations that limit the number of hours that residents may work within a week and that require residency programs in every discipline to restructure call schedules and expectations. This change is a reaction to concerns that overly fatigued residents are compromising patient care. As programs struggle to adapt to these new standards, it is worthwhile to reflect on the higher ethical imperative to care for professionals as well as patients by setting more realistic limits. It is hoped that this change, once it is processed, will be the beginning of a shift away from the unhealthy traditions of the past toward a new era in which the health of health care professionals during and after training is more highly valued.

Case Scenarios

A 34-year-old resident becomes distressed after the suicide of one of her patients. She experiences persistent feelings of failure, has difficulty sleeping, and becomes afraid of being "fired" despite multiple evaluations documenting her excellent performance in the program. She increasingly uses alcohol to help her sleep.

A 39-year-old psychiatrist becomes romantically involved with a patient seen on one occasion in the emergency room. "We were both getting over a divorce, and we had a lot in common," he told his supervisor. "She was never really my patient, because I was just a consultant on the case."

■ REFERENCES

Accreditation Council for Graduate Medical Education: Proposed Duty Hour Standards in the Program and Institutional Requirements for Review and Comment. Chicago, IL, Accreditation Council for Graduate Medical Education, 2002

Council on Scientific Affairs: Results and implications of the AMA–APA Physician Mortality Project. Stage II. JAMA 257:2949–2953, 1987

Grosch WN, Olsen DC: When Helping Starts to Hurt: A New Look at Burnout Among Psychotherapists. New York, WW Norton, 1994

Kohut H: Analysis of the Self. New York, International Universities Press, 1981

Kohut H: How Does Analysis Cure? Chicago, IL, University of Chicago Press, 1984

Miller MN, McGowen RK: The painful truth: physicians are not invincible. South Med J 93:966–973, 2000

Physician suicide. JAMA 258:1607, 1987

Roberts LW, Warner TD, Carter D, et al: Caring for medical students as patients: access to services and care-seeking practices of 1,027 students at nine medical schools. Collaborative Research Group on Medical Student Healthcare. Acad Med 75:272–277, 2000

Roberts LW, Warner TD, Lyketsos C, et al: Perceptions of academic vulnerability associated with personal illness: a study of 1,027 students at nine medical schools. Collaborative Research Group on Medical Student Health. Compr Psychiatry 42:1–15, 2001

Sargent DA: Preventing physician suicide. JAMA 257:2955–2956, 1987

Sotile MO, Sotile WM: The Medical Marriage: A Couple's Survival Guide. New York, Carol Publishing, 1996

Stoudemire A, Rhoads JM: When the doctor needs a doctor: special considerations for the physician-patient. Ann Intern Med 98(5 pt 1):654–659, 1983

Winnicott DW: The Child, the Family, and the Outside World. London, Penguin, 1964

ETHICAL ISSUES IN CLINICAL TRAINING

Physicians in training, both medical students and residents, face unique ethical challenges as they acquire the knowledge and skills that will allow them to care for suffering human beings competently and compassionately. Each stage of training represents different ethical tasks and dilemmas which, if successfully mastered, lead to the attainment of a higher level of ethical sensitivity and professional responsibility. It is essential that supervisors and educators be attuned and attentive to these developmental stages of ethical growth so that they may intentionally create opportunities to foster self-awareness, habits of self-care, and humanistic and empathic patient–physician relationships. This is indeed necessary if clinical education is to be more than "on the job" training at best and exhausting, traumatic, and cynicism-engendering labor at worst. In psychiatric training, appropriate didactic and experiential teaching, mentoring, and support can assist in preserving the moral foundation of the profession of psychiatry and can help build optimal ethical knowledge, skills, and attitudes of these physicians who dedicate their careers to the care of mentally ill individuals.

Education leaders increasingly are making explicit their commitment to the moral foundation of clinical medicine. The Association of American Medical Colleges in 1998 developed a formal set of recommendations regarding the learning objectives for medical student education. These objectives centered on the following premises: 1) physicians must be altruistic; 2) physicians must be knowledgeable; 3) physicians must be skillful; and 4) physicians must be dutiful (American Association of Medical Colleges 1998). The American Psychiatric Association has recommended that ethics training for psychiatry residents encompass several key content, skill, and attitude domains, as presented in Table 15–1. The Accreditation Council for Graduate Medical Education (2003) recently implemented clearer and more rigorous standards for residency programs regarding the evaluation of resident competence, including the related areas of ethics, professionalism, and communication skills.

TABLE 15–1. **Model curriculum for psychiatric training recommended by the American Psychiatric Association**

Knowledge

Existence of overlaps and differences between legal and ethical issues and how to access relevant laws

Importance and history of ethical codes to the profession of medicine and how the principles continue to apply to evolving situations

Basic philosophical principles, such as paternalism, autonomy, beneficence, nonmaleficence, and justice, which can be used to analyze ethical conflicts

The content of *The Principles of Medical Ethics With Annotations Especially Applicable to Psychiatry* and the practical meaning and application of each section

    Competent and respectful treatment

    Honest dealing and disclosure

    Respect for the law

    Respect for confidences and colleagues

    Commitment to study and obtain consultation

    Practice environment and terminating treatment

    Improving the community and relationships with government

Skills

Provide competent psychiatry evaluation and treatment

Avoid boundary violations with patients and colleagues

Avoid sexual exploitation of patients and colleagues

Preserve patient confidentiality

Evaluate and manage suicidal patients

| TABLE 15–1. | **Model curriculum for psychiatric training recommended by the American Psychiatric Association *(continued)*** |

Evaluate and manage homicidal patients

Obtain and use proxy decisions from patients

Institute involuntary commitment

Manage patient treatment refusal

Relate professionally and ethically with colleagues, faculty, and supervisors

Recognize and resolve competing ethical interests

Recognize legal obligations

Recognize the limits of one's own abilities and seek consultation when necessary

Recognize and intervene with impaired or unethical colleagues

Apply ethical principles to consultation for medical colleagues or the courts

Admit and discharge patients

Participate in utilization review and peer review

Bill for psychiatric services

Attitudes

Compassion and honest dealing with patients and colleagues

Respect for human dignity

Respect for the law

Respect for the rights and confidences of patients, colleagues, and other health professionals

Commitment to providing competent medical service to patients

Commitment to one's own continued professional development

Commitment to improving the profession and the community

■ SPECIAL ETHICAL CHALLENGES OF CLINICAL TRAINING

Clinical trainees inhabit three ethically important roles: as students, as trainees within the profession of medicine, and as early career caregivers within a specialty area. These three roles each have inherent ethical imperatives. The three roles have much in common. For example, they all value truth telling, promise keeping, and honest dealings with others. They all value respect, effort, and diligence. The three roles are nevertheless distinct, and their differences may create conflicts from time to time for clinicians in training. For instance, the student's responsibility is to learn, whereas the clinician's responsibility is to provide an optimal—or at least appropriate—standard of care to patients. When one is learning to be a clinical professional, it is inevitable that mistakes will occur. People with mental illness may be vulnerable and unable to advocate for themselves in clinical situations in which mistakes take place. These considerations are very important, especially in the context of caring for individuals with diminished interpersonal power (e.g., institutionalized persons; ill children or elderly persons; seriously mentally ill adults; individuals with diminished societal power and roles, such as mentally ill undocumented immigrants). In essence, the roles of early career professionals learning to care for people with mental illness carry ethical imperatives and tensions, some of which are unique to the developmental situation of training and many of which will accompany trainees throughout their professional lives.

Clinical training thus presents predictable and developmentally necessary ethical challenges. We will highlight four. First, clinical trainees carry enormous patient care responsibilities during a period in which they are not yet fully clinically competent. On inpatient rotations, medical students and residents perform psychiatric evaluations and physical examinations for large numbers of patients. In emergency rooms, interns and residents are often the ones to decide whether an intoxicated patient who is threatening suicide but who refuses hospitalization is allowed to leave the facility. Similarly, how grave does "grave passive neglect" need to be for a person with psychosis and poor self-care to be admitted involuntarily to the psychiatric unit? Does an elderly patient with early dementia need a treatment guardian to make medication decisions? Should a report be filed with child protective services when an adolescent offhandedly mentions that his mom is "on drugs" and is "never around." In some settings, the clinical trainee may be the only person with any advanced mental health training to actually *see* the patient. Although the trainee receives supervision from an attending physician or a more senior team member on such cases, these decisions often ride solely on the trainee's history taking, mental status examination, and assessment, as well as on his or her "hunches," which may or may not be well attuned to the complexities of the patient's clinical presentation.

Second, clinical education inherently involves an ethical conflict. "Being in training" means "learning on people," which is not a comfortable thought for individuals who are sensitive to the ethical meaning of the training experience. In surgery or medicine, this necessary learning process may mean performing procedures on ill individuals, without much preparation ("see one, do one, teach one"). There must always be a first time one "sets" a fractured bone, gathers an arterial blood sample, sutures a wound, or detects (or not) a serious pathological murmur. In psychiatric training, there are dozens of judgment errors—big and small, omission and commission—a fledgling clinician may make. Errors may occur as a trainee learns psychotherapy skills by conducting psychotherapy with a depressed or traumatized patient or as a resident learns appropriate medication dosing by treating a frail mentally ill elderly patient. Trainees who are not yet prepared for the complicated, nuanced clinical and ethical aspects of decisional capacity assessments are nonetheless confronted with the necessity to perform such assessments from the first week of residency, when they may be required to appear in court for a patient's involuntary commitment hearing. Often, the greater risk of error is balanced by the extra thoroughness and care that trainees give to their patients and to their work, but the consequences of error can be serious, ranging from medication side effects to unanticipated suicide attempts.

Third, clinical trainees often must do things that they find alien, uncomfortable, or culturally "wrong" in caring for people with mental illness. The range of possibilities is broad—from asking a patient about the intimate details of her sexual history and behaviors to taking away a patient's personal liberty by involuntarily committing him to psychiatric treatment, from turning away a patient with mental health needs because of lack of insurance to caring for a patient who exhibits beliefs and violent behaviors that are disquieting, from giving a medication because it is "on formulary" to withholding valuable treatment because of legal imperatives. This is a difficult aspect of the newly acquired clinical role.

Interestingly, learning to provide mental health care means paying attention to one's inner sense of things. In learning to become a health care professional, one's principal instrument is the self. The clinical trainee is thus encouraged to shut off certain insights while attending to others. For these reasons, the educational experience involves moments that feel, at best, uneasy and confusing and, at worst, coercive and painful.

A fourth ethical challenge in preparing trainees to care for people with mental illness pertains to stress and self-care during the training process. More than other clinical specialty areas, the mental health professions clearly recognize the importance of clinicians themselves being psychologically sound and emotionally resilient and engaging in appropriate self-care as necessary to be able to provide mental health care to others. The irony, of course, is that the training process is exhausting and demanding, leaving little time or energy for the clinical trainee to pursue healthy and emotionally sustaining activities. The combination of heavy workload, sleep deprivation, and academic, clinical, and personal obligations can render even the most psychologically healthy resident vulnerable to stress. Indeed, trainees are at significant risk for mental health, addiction, and some physical health issues by virtue of the rigors of their educational preparation (Hughes et al. 1991; Jex et al. 1992; Roberts et al. 2000). Simply witnessing the suffering of mentally ill people generates pain within a mental health trainee; beyond this fact of professional work, within mental health care some programs are experienced as unkind or overtly abusive toward their trainees. Even in the most humane programs, faculty supervisors may become stressed and overwhelmed, providing poor role models for their early career colleagues. The message of training is thus an ambiguous, conflicted one, conveying superhuman, or perhaps inhuman, expectations. From an ethical perspective, these conditions are critically important, because, as described in Chapter 1, being self-reflective and nondefensive is essential to the process of sound ethical decision making. Furthermore, decades of conceptual and empirical work suggest that the clinical training process is one that too often inculcates cynicism and diminishment of the self rather than imparting ideals of the profession and affirmation of the self in preparing trainees to help alleviate the suffering of others.

■ EMPIRICAL STUDIES ON ETHICS AND CLINICAL TRAINING

Many empirical studies have been performed on ethics and ethics instruction in clinical education. A uniform finding has been the strong interest of clinical trainees in patient care ethics and the desire for more substantive preparation for the ethical aspects of clinical care responsibilities. For example, Jacobson et al. (1989) surveyed 202 internal medicine residents at three training programs, finding that a majority wanted more training on ethics-related topics. In an analogous study, Roberts et al. (1996) performed a survey with 181 psychiatry residents in 10 training programs in the United States. Seventy-six percent reported that they had encountered an ethical dilemma for which they felt unprepared, and 92% reported that ethics training had been useful in helping them respond to ethical dilemmas arising with patients. One-third reported receiving no ethics preparation during medical school, and 46% reported receiving none in residency. Between 24% and 75% of the residents expressed the belief that more curricular attention should be given to ethics-related topics (Roberts et al. 1996). Coverdale et al. (1992) found similar results in their 1992 study of 121 psychiatry chief residents and program directors, which revealed that although 40% of the programs had no formal ethics curriculum, the trainees expressed enthusiasm for additional ethics teaching.

More recently, Roberts and colleagues (in press) performed an ethics education study with 336 medical students and residents at the University of New Mexico. We found that the trainees in this study strongly endorsed the importance of professionalism among physicians, the prevalence of ethical conflicts in everyday practice, and the perception that ethics training is helpful in resolving ethical conflicts. They also identified the goals of ethics preparation as improving patient care and clinical decision making, gaining a better recognition of ethics issues, developing interpersonal skills useful in resolving ethics conflicts, learning strategies for clarifying values-laden choices, and acquiring a working knowledge of social science, philosophy, religion, and the law as they apply to clinical care. Similar to findings of other studies, clinically oriented learning approaches overall were perceived as far superior to more isolated or less relevant approaches, and formal assessment of ethics skills was seen as acceptable and appropriate.

All of these studies have revealed the beneficial impact of positive role models and direct involvement of clinicians in patient care and the importance of teaching methods that are integrated into clinical and supervisory routines of training. They also suggest differential interest and commitment to ethics education by students of different backgrounds and attributes. Women trainees have consistently shown greater interest and more diverse learning preferences than their male counterparts, and interest in specific topics appears to be driven largely by the unique demands and nature of clinical specialty areas.

The failure of the educational system to provide sufficient ethics training is worrisome in light of empirical evidence suggesting that clinical education has a detrimental effect on the humanistic values and attitudes of trainees and their overall well-being. The effects of this lack of ethics training were explored in an anonymous written survey of 665 third- and fourth-year medical students conducted by Feudtner et al. (1994). In this study, 58% of the students reported that they had done something they felt was unethical, 52% had misled a patient, 61% had witnessed unethical behavior in medical team members, and 67% felt bad about something they had done as clinical clerks. Importantly, the majority of the medical students (62%) reported that at least some of their ethical principles had declined since they entered training and that fear of a poor evaluation by a supervisor was a coercive pressure that led to improper conduct. Similarly, in a survey of 571 second-year residents conducted by Baldwin et al. (1998), three-quarters reported having directly observed patient mistreatment and colleagues working in an impaired condition. More than one-quarter of the residents stated that they had been forced to do something unethical or immoral during the prior year.

In terms of resident well-being, Bellini and colleagues (2002) examined variations in mood and empathy in 61 residents longitudinally across their internship year. These physicians in training started the year with less anger, tension, fatigue, depression, and confusion and more vigor relative to the general or college population, and they exhibited better empathy and less personal distress than did comparison subjects. After 5 months of internship, however, scores on depression–dejection, anger–hostility, fatigue–inertia, and personal distress scales had risen, with a corresponding decrease in vigor–activity and empathy ratings. The changes persisted during the remainder of the internship year. Hughes et al. (1992) examined patterns of substance abuse in residents according to specialty, finding that psychiatry and emergency medicine residents showed higher rates of substance abuse than did residents in all other specialties. A study conducted by Firth-Cozens (1987) examined the relationship between burnout and patient care among 115 internal medicine residents. Three-quarters of the responding residents met criteria for exhaustion ("burnout"), and 53% of these reported an episode of suboptimal patient care at least monthly (versus 21% of residents without such emotional and physical depletion). The factor most strongly associated with burnout and resultant poor care was feeling diminished and depersonalized in the training environment.

Less discouraging are the studies of the positive impact of ethics-related educational interventions in clinical training. Clinically relevant educational activities appear to improve the sensitivity and competence exhibited and the confidence felt by trainees as they respond to ethical problems. Gann et al. (1991) conducted a single, brief, intensive workshop on AIDS for 187 medical students and found over 3 consecutive years that students' knowledge and attitudes improved on important practice measures. Green et al. (1995) found a significant increase in ethical awareness as measured by the

Toronto Ethical Sensitivity Instrument in medical students after a single workshop on psychiatric ethics. Junek et al. (1979) and Scheidt et al. (1986) used videotaped patient interactions to examine interviewing skills and found that providing feedback to medical trainees enhanced their empathy and communication skills. Similarly, Ende et al. (1986) performed an observational cohort study of interviewing skills with 11 pairs of interns and faculty. All interactions were videotaped and transcribed. It was found that feedback and communication from preceptors enhanced the interns' self-esteem and sense of moral responsibility.

In other studies, Siegler et al. (1982) found that junior medical students demonstrated increased reflectiveness regarding ethical decisions after participating in a 12- to 14-hour clinical ethics seminar on the general medicine unit focusing on the students' own patient cases. Bebeau and Thoma (1994) found statistically significant increases in moral reasoning, as measured by the Defining Issues Test (DIT), in 7 out of 8 consecutive classes of dental students that participated in a problem-oriented dental ethics curriculum. Many other investigators have had similar results with the DIT throughout the allied health sciences (Self et al. 1998). Lo and Schroeder (1981), using a quasi-experimental prospective design in which they served as participant-observers on medical rounds, found an increase (from 3.9% to 17%) in residents' accurate identification of ethical problems in patient cases after the intervention. Sulmasy et al. (1994) assessed the long-term clinical impact of a broad-based ethics education program on resident DNR (do not resuscitate) orders and found significant improvement in documentation with respect to 11 concurrent care concerns (e.g., ranging from the spiritual needs of patients to the clinical appropriateness of pressor medications and adjustment of pain medications). Sulmasy et al. (1990) also conducted a 1-year randomized trial to assess the impact of an ethics curriculum on the knowledge, confidence, and responses of 85 residents, with an emphasis on end-of-life care. One-quarter of the residents underwent a lecture series, 25% underwent a lecture series combined with clinical case conferences with an ethicist in attendance, and 50% served as controls. Although formal knowledge of ethics did not differ among the three groups, confidence regarding identifying and acting on ethical issues was significantly greater in the experimental groups. These findings suggest the beneficial impact of ethics-related educational interventions that focus on practical, "real life" issues encountered by trainees as they provide patient care (Sulmasy et al. 1990). Finally, Roberts has performed evaluations of the ethical skill competence of medical students in formal standardized patient interactions—for example, in obtaining informed consent for a recommended HIV test. This work has revealed the feasibility of implementing valid and student-accepted measures for evaluating ethics competence and strong skill levels among graduating medical students at our institution (Carter and Roberts 1997).

■ EDUCATIONAL STRATEGIES FOR ETHICS EDUCATION IN CLINICAL TRAINING

Effective preparation for the ethical and professional aspects of caring for mentally ill individuals will have several characteristics: it should be developmentally attuned and ecologically sound, naturally evolving from the structure and realities of psychiatric training. It should not be treated as an "add on" topic. In terms of curricular content, the American Psychiatric Association has offered specific recommendations for topics to be covered in resident ethics curricula (see Table 15–1 earlier in this chapter). Recommendations for ethics teaching in clinical training are outlined in Table 15–2, and goals and objectives of such training are listed in Table 15–3. A method for teaching ethics through psychiatric supervision is outlined in Table 15–4. Experience in ethics teaching and empirical evidence suggest the important contribution of role models, consultants, and innovative and integrated methods. Finally, ethics education in clinical training should be explicitly evaluated, not only in the sense of how well the trainees enjoyed the curriculum but also in regard to how well it imparted clinically important ethics skills.

TABLE 15–2. **Recommendations for clinical ethics teaching in clinical training**

Design curricula that address clinically relevant issues in mental health ethics, including confidentiality, informed consent, decisional capacity, and commitment

Develop special events that highlight the importance and value of ethics (e.g., grand rounds, invited visiting professors, evidence-based ethics research presentations)

Create diverse contexts for learning and self-reflection and draw out the ethical meaning within routine clinical situations

Find ways to provide additional educational opportunities for trainees who have a greater interest in ethics topics and skills

Respectfully and sensitively guide trainees in identifying their own responses and defenses in relation to clinical ethical issues

Provide access to ethics resources and encourage the use of colleagues, supervisors, and expert consultants in addressing ethically complex situations

Encourage faculty mentors with an interest in ethics to obtain formal training and to provide time and resources to support ethics teaching for trainees

Include ethics knowledge and skill and professional attitudes in the formal evaluation of trainees

Help trainees as they deal constructively with their own limitations and errors; without losing sight of clinical competence standards, work with trainees to perceive mistakes and bad-outcome situations as unfortunate but as offering formative lessons

Seek opportunities for trainees to discuss the stresses of training and their impact on patient care activities, including ethically important decision making

---

TABLE 15–3. **Goals and objectives for ethics education**

Early in clinical training:

- Ability to *define and use ethics terms* accurately
- Ability to *identify values-laden aspects and ethical considerations* present in a clinical care situation
- Ability to *apply ethics principles to understand and select among different ethically sound approaches* to clinical care situations
- Ability to *perform literature searches on ethics topics* related to issues present in clinical care situations
- Ability to *recognize the limits of one's personal knowledge and role* in a clinical care situation
- Ability to *utilize clinical information, ethics guidelines, and empirical evidence in clarifying ethical questions*
- Ability to *observe and characterize a clinical interaction* and then to *identify how factors in the interaction may affect the ethical dimensions of the patient's care*
- Ability to *describe and reflect upon one's own professional training experiences* within the context of professional attitudes, values, and ethics

Later in clinical training, demonstrable mastery of the above, plus:

- Ability to *assess more sophisticated, complex clinical care situations* in light of clinical, ethical, psychosocial, and legal issues
- Ability to *identify, assess, and anticipate sequelae for different approaches* to more sophisticated, complex clinical care situations in light of clinical, ethical, psychosocial, and legal issues
- Ability to *demonstrate appropriate self-directed learning and growth in ethics and professionalism*
- Ability to *apply formal ethical decision-making models to ethically complex situations*

In preparation for the transition to independent clinical practice, demonstrable mastery of the above, plus:

- Ability to *identify and respond to subtle clinical, ethical, psychosocial, and legal issues* present in a clinical care situation

Ability to *perform key ethically important clinical tasks* (e.g., obtaining informed consent or refusal for care, safeguarding confidentiality, addressing stigmatizing health issues) in a manner that reflects sensitivity, demonstrates awareness of ethical complexities present in the situation, and fulfills accepted standards of care

TABLE 15–3. **Goals and objectives for ethics education**
              (continued)

In preparation for the transition to independent clinical practice, demonstrable mastery of the above, plus *(continued)***:**

- Ability to *identify a course of action that employs advanced clinical ethics problem-resolution techniques* (e.g., recognizing the limits of one's knowledge, pursuing additional data gathering, seeking collaboration and consultation with individuals with cross-disciplinary expertise, such as law, medical subspecialties)
- Ability to reflect upon one's own professional training experiences, to characterize how one's own value system may influence one's clinical practices, and to safeguard against one's personal biases

TABLE 15–4. **Strategies for implementing ethics in clinical supervision**

Help the resident to define the clinical aspects of the patient's case.

Guide the resident in the identification of ethical issues and conflicts in the clinical situation, while giving him or her an opportunity to describe personal thoughts and concerns relating to the case.

Collaborate with the resident in gathering information and necessary clinical and ethical expertise.

Explore possible responses to the clinical and ethical problems with the resident, deciding what acceptable choices exist and anticipating the outcomes of these possible decisions.

Provide guidance and support as the resident implements the decision

Create a context for reflection and review.

Case Scenarios

The medical director of a community health center calls a second-year resident into his office to tell her that a patient she evaluated in the emergency room one night 8 months ago has killed himself.

A second-year resident states that she will not "do shock therapy" on patients, even if it is a program requirement that she learn this clinical treatment procedure.

An intern becomes upset during inpatient rounds when she is chastised by teammates for admitting a patient the night before and for giving a pass to a personality disordered patient.

An intern with anorexia nervosa seeks psychiatric care for a relapse precipitated by the stresses of training. She learns that the only eating disorder specialist is her residency program director.

A young faculty attending physician at a psychiatric hospital is working 14-hour days and on weekends. He is irritable toward patients, his teammates, and his family. He repeatedly fails to show up for his supervision sessions with the residents. He is having trouble sleeping, ignores his children, and has stopped exercising and pursuing his hobbies.

A patient asks a resident to write a prescription for a medication at twice the recommended dose, so that he will be able to stretch the pills over a longer period of time and pay less money out of pocket at the pharmacy.

A resident at an intake clinic is encouraged to record a different diagnosis on the billing sheet because it "pays."

■ REFERENCES

Accreditation Council for Graduate Medical Education: ACGME duty hours standards now in effect for all residency programs. July 1, 2003. Available at: http://www.acgme.org. Accessed December 12, 2003

American Association of Medical Colleges: Medical School Objectives Project. Washington, DC, American Association of Medical Colleges, 1998

Baldwin DC Jr, Daugherty SR, Rowley BD: Unethical and unprofessional conduct observed by residents during their first year of training. Acad Med 73:1195–1200, 1998

Bebeau MJ, Thoma SJ: The impact of a dental ethics curriculum on moral reasoning. J Dent Educ 58:684–692, 1994

Bellini LM, Baime M, Shea JA: Variation of mood and empathy during internship. JAMA 287:3143–3146, 2002

Carter D, Roberts LW: Medical students' attitudes toward patients with HIV infection. A comparison study of 169 first-year students at the University of Chicago and the University of New Mexico. Journal of the Gay and Lesbian Medical Association 1(4):209–226, 1997

Coverdale JH, Bayer T, Isbell P, et al: Are we teaching psychiatrists to be ethical? Acad Psychiatry 16:199–205, 1992

Ende J, Pozen JT, Levinsky NG: Enhancing learning during a clinical clerkship: the value of a structured curriculum. J Gen Intern Med 1:232–237, 1986

Feudtner C, Christakis DA, Christakis NA: Do clinical clerks suffer ethical erosion? Students' perceptions of their ethical environment and personal development. Acad Med 69:670–679, 1994

Firth-Cozens J: Emotional distress in junior house officers. BMJ (Clin Res Ed) 295:533–536, 1987

Gann PH, Anderson S, Regan MB: Shifts in medical student beliefs about AIDS after a comprehensive training experience. Am J Prev Med 7:172–177, 1991

Green B, Miller PD, Routh CP: Teaching ethics in psychiatry: a one-day workshop for clinical students. J Med Ethics 21:234–238, 1995

Hughes PH, Conard SE, Baldwin DC Jr, et al: Resident physician substance use in the United States. JAMA 265:2069–2073, 1991

Hughes PH, Baldwin DC Jr, Sheehan DV, et al: Resident physician substance use, by specialty. Am J Psychiatry 149:1348–1354, 1992

Jacobson JA, Tolle SW, Stocking C, et al: Internal medicine residents' preferences regarding medical ethics education. Acad Med 64:760–764, 1989

Jex SM, Hughes P, Storr C, et al: Relations among stressors, strains, and substance use among resident physicians. Int J Addict 27:979–994, 1992

Junek W, Burra P, Leichner P: Teaching interviewing skills by encountering patients. J Med Educ 54:402–407, 1979

Lo B, Schroeder SA: Frequency of ethical dilemmas in a medical inpatient service. Arch Intern Med 141:1062–1064, 1981

Roberts LW, McCarty T, Lyketsos C, et al: What and how psychiatry residents at ten training programs wish to learn ethics. Acad Psychiatry 20:131–143, 1996

Roberts LW, Warner TD, Carter D, et al: Caring for medical students as patients: access to services and care-seeking practices of 1,027 students at nine medical schools. Collaborative Research Group on Medical Student Healthcare. Acad Med 75:272–277, 2000

Roberts LW, Green Hammond KA, Geppert C, et al: The positive role of professionalism and ethics training in medical education: a comparison of medical student and resident perspectives. Acad Psychiatry (in press)

Scheidt PC, Lazoritz S, Ebbeling WL, et al: Evaluation of system providing feedback to students on videotaped patient encounters. J Med Educ 61:585–590, 1986

Self DJ, Olivarez M, Baldwin DC Jr: The amount of small-group case-study discussion needed to improve moral reasoning skills of medical students. Acad Med 73:521–523, 1998

Siegler M, Rezler AG, Connell KJ: Using simulated case studies to evaluate a clinical ethics course for junior students. J Med Educ 57:380–385, 1982

Sulmasy DP, Geller G, Levine DM, et al: Medical house officers' knowledge, attitudes, and confidence regarding medical ethics. Arch Intern Med 150:2509–2513, 1990

Sulmasy DP, Terry PB, Faden RR, et al: Long-term effects of ethics education on the quality of care for patients who have do-not-resuscitate orders [see comments]. J Gen Intern Med 9:622–626, 1994

ETHICAL ISSUES IN PSYCHIATRIC RESEARCH

Three ethics principles govern human research: 1) *respect for persons,* honoring the dignity and promoting the autonomy of research participants; 2) *beneficence,* the duty to seek maximal good and to do minimal harm through the conduct of research; and 3) *justice,* ensuring that the segment of the population bearing the greatest burden for research also benefit from it and ensuring that special groups are not exploited as a result of individual, interpersonal, or societal attributes or powerlessness. These bioethics principles were most elegantly and clearly articulated in the 1979 landmark *Belmont Report* and are echoed throughout other historic research ethics documents (Table 16–1) (National Commission for the Protection of Human Subjects of Biomedical and Behavioral Research 1979).

Ethically sound research embraces the three principles of *respect for persons, beneficence,* and *justice* and translates them into practice through the design, methods, and safeguards of experimental protocols. Ethically sound research hinges on the expertise and integrity of investigators and the absence of significant conflicts of interest that might threaten objectivity, decisions, and/or actions. Moreover, it seeks to advance the concerns and well-being of special groups and potentially vulnerable populations, such as the mentally ill, children, the elderly, the dying, the captive, and others. Finally, specific guidelines have been developed with respect to animal research, including experimentation potentially related to psychiatric investigation.

TABLE 16–1. **History of the Common Rule**

Year	Title	Summary
1974	National Research Act	Codified DHEW Moratorium on federally funded fetal research IRB review of human research for DHEW funds
1974–1978	National Commission for Protection of Human Subjects of Biomedical and Behavioral Research	Reports on research involving special populations; regulatory guidance for IRBs, informed consent *Belmont Report* outlining ethical principles in protecting human subjects in research
1978	Revised DHEW	Regulations protecting pregnant women, fetuses, prisoners, and in vitro fertilization
1980–1983	President's Commission for the Study of Ethical Problems in Medicine and Biomedical and Behavioral Research	Reviewed federal policies governing human research Recommended that all federal agencies adopt DHHS (DHEW) regulations for the protection of subjects
1981	Revision of DHHS	IRB responsibilities and procedures FDA regulations revised to correspond to DHHS
1982	President's Science Advisor/Office of Science and Technology	Appointed to head interagency committee to develop a common policy for protection of human research subjects
1983	DHHS regulation	Protections governing children in research

TABLE 16–1. **History of the Common Rule** *(continued)*

Year	Title	Summary
1991	Final Common Federal Policy: the "Common Rule"	Regulations for 15 federal agencies regarding human subject protection were combined via executive order
		Identical to basic DHHS policy for protection of research subjects
		Additional protections for pregnant women, fetuses, in vitro fertilization, prisoners, children
		FDA informed consent and IRB regulations changed to meet these standards

Note. CIA=U.S. Central Intelligence Agency; DHEW=U.S. Department of Health, Education, and Welfare; DHHS= U.S. Department of Health and Human Services; FDA=U.S. Food and Drug Administration; IRB=institutional review board.

■ DESIGN, METHODS, AND THE NEED FOR ETHICS SAFEGUARDS

Ethics and scientific design issues fit closely together in three key respects. First, it is widely accepted that a study's design should be based on a research question that is valuable, significant, timely, and justified, and that the study's methods should test hypotheses in a manner that will produce meaningful, interpretable results. Concretely, the design and methods must be appropriate to prove or disprove the study's hypotheses. Otherwise, because of the principle of *respect for persons* and its underlying philosophical basis, it is not acceptable to include human beings as "objects" of study in research that lacks potential for a true scientific contribution and a greater social good. Second, an ethically sound study will employ a design and procedures that minimize risks to study participants. In essence, an experiment must not expose individuals to greater levels of risk than are necessary to ask its underlying scientific question. For this reason, an experiment should not use a relatively more risky design when a relatively less risky alternative design will suffice scientifically. Finally, the scientific design and its interventions should not be so complex that they cannot be understood and their intent and ramifications appreciated by individuals who are considering participation in the study (Roberts 1998).

Various experimental designs have become the subject of controversy as scientific methods have evolved and awareness of ethical issues in research has increased. Recently, studies that entail placebo trials, medication washout periods, or symptom challenge maneuvers have raised difficult questions regarding their scientific necessity and true risks. Conceptual arguments have been developed both for and against these designs, yet few data are available on the personal and scientific impact of these approaches and their alternatives to help clarify the concerns surrounding them. For example, it is not known whether individuals who participate in placebo studies ultimately have worse outcomes than those who participate in other types of experiments or than patients who have never been in research protocols. Eventually, controversial or problematic designs may be discarded as they become scientifically obsolete or, alternatively, special methodological approaches will arise around them to ensure that they are conducted ethically.

This latter process of building additional ethical safeguards has occurred with deception studies in the field of behavioral science. Deception studies, in general, are intended to explore phenomena in which awareness of the focus of the experiment will impair the ability to collect accurate data. A deception study can meet current ethical standards if it explores nonstigmatizing phenomena, involves participants who have consented to the possibility of deception in the protocol, and provides an appropriate "debriefing" to participants at the conclusion of their involvement in the study. The issues are similar in biomedical research designs that use "deception"—that is, incomplete disclosure of the specific interventions that the participant will experience. For example, in a medication trial employing a "double blind" design in which neither the investigator nor the participant knows which medication is being administered, it is possible to differentiate psychological (e.g., attitudinal) influences of the researchers and the participants from the "true" effects of the medications being studied. However, notorious, ethically disturbing psychological deception experiments have been conducted, such as studies of personal and sexual behaviors in which investigators did not appreciate the ethical ramifications of not informing or of outrightly deceiving participants. Such experiments have been experienced by participants and recognized by the scientific community as inordinately intrusive and exploitative. Consequently, special steps to ensure the ethical conduct of deception studies have been created and agreed upon within the fields of behavioral and biomedical science. These steps include an informed consent process that is broad enough to encompass the material actually being assessed within the study; recruitment of participants with sound decisional capabilities, given the object of the exploration; special sensitivity and efforts to minimize embarrassment or discomfort should these arise for participants; and appropriate debriefing at the end of each participant's study involvement. Similar ethically oriented methods may be employed to enhance the ethical protections around study participants in experiments whose designs pose special problems.

In sum, it is natural that certain experimental designs will undergo careful scrutiny as scientific designs and methods advance. The fact that such questions arise should be viewed not as a failure of the science, but rather as a scientific "success" in that investigators are openly accountable, self-observing, and thoughtful about the justification for their experimental methods. The key is to accurately assess the scientific necessity of and the alternatives to the design, to determine the potential risks to participants, and to collaborate with others to review these issues and develop additional ways of improving the ethical features of the design wherever possible.

■ ETHICS SAFEGUARDS

Several safeguards are built into the process of *all* biomedical experimentation to offer ethical protection to human participants. These safeguards are implemented at the level of the institution (e.g., medical center, source of funding) and the individual investigator, and they are codified and enforced through federal regulations (e.g., Office for Protection From Research Risks). The most critical of these safeguards include 1) institutional review boards (IRBs); 2) informed consent; 3) advance, alternative, and collaborative decision making; 4) additional expert and peer review processes; and 5) confidentiality protections. Each of these safeguards is discussed below in light of its theoretical basis and empirical support (Roberts et al. 2001).

Institutional Review and Data and Safety Monitoring

IRBs prospectively review human and animal research occurring in the institutional context. Their aim is twofold: to ensure scientific merit and to ensure that study participants are treated ethically and that their "rights and welfare" are protected. IRBs are empowered to approve, to insist on modifications and revisions as a condition of approval, or to disapprove research before it is undertaken. Their decisions carry weight outside the institution as well, because most funding agencies will require IRB approval before providing support for projects. Although the procedures of IRBs primarily focus on protocols prospectively (e.g., reviewing consent forms for their adequacy, examining the scientific rationale for the experiment), IRBs have responsibility for the ongoing monitoring of research within the institution. The IRB can stop research, even after it has been approved, that is found to be conducted incompetently, is discovered to be performed significantly differently than originally described, or is determined to pose inordinate risks to participants (Levine 1986).

IRBs are constituted to combine both expertise and representation. IRB members should be knowledgeable about both scientific issues and ethics protections, including the content of relevant regulations and literature. IRB membership should also allow for adequate representation of the viewpoints of potential research participants. For example, it has long been recognized that both genders, nonscientists, and community representatives should be included on IRB committees. More recently, it has been proposed that people deriving from special groups, such as individuals with mental illness, should be included as voting members of IRBs. Greater diversity of perspectives and broader collaboration serve as the rationale for IRB membership constituted in this way.

The actual functioning of IRBs has been poorly understood, and often IRBs are provided insufficient resources, given their critical role within biomedical and other research institutions. For example, the "cultures" and actual procedures of individual IRBs may vary significantly according to the nature of the institution, the region of the country, and the kind of research most frequently reviewed. IRBs may "delegate" significant portions of their work to other elements of the institution, for example, by asking for the scientific review prior to IRB submission (e.g., through a departmental review process), which may result in less objective scrutiny of proposals. In addition, IRB members are not required to have formal preparation, and they commonly are "volunteers" who accept IRB duties in addition to their usual responsibilities. Finally, IRBs often may not receive adequate support (e.g., administrative staff, budget, space) to perform anything but the most basic prospective review and annual review activities. Some poorly implemented and some competent but overburdened IRBs have been faulted for inadequate review processes. Under more optimal circumstances, efforts to improve education of IRB members and investigators, to conduct intermittent monitoring of certain protocols, to work more closely with communities and special groups, and to develop explicit policies and standards related to research might be possible.

Informed Consent

The doctrine of informed consent requires that all individuals truly understand and freely make choices about "intrusions" upon their physical and psychological selves. As in informed consent for clinical care (see Chapter 4), informed consent for participation in research is a process, not a single event, and ideally occurs within the context of a professional relationship characterized by trust and integrity. Research consent, also like clinical consent, entails three elements: information sharing, decisional capacity, and voluntarism.

Information Sharing

Research consent involves accurate and complete information regarding the reason for and nature of the proposed intervention, its associated biological and psychosocial risks and their magnitude, its associated biological and psychosocial benefits and their magnitude, the alternatives (including no intervention at all), who is responsible for the research, and other ramifications (e.g., economic or social consequences) of participation. The sharing of this information reflects respect for the individual and respect for the truth. Outside of the very specific situation of emergency research consent, this information should be imparted in a manner that is clear, that is not rushed, and that promotes the genuine understanding of the potential participant. For complex or risky protocols, it is important, then, that disclosure associated with consent occur on at least two occasions and that supplementary materials (e.g., pamphlets or even videotapes) be provided.

Decisional Capacity

An individual who is invited to enroll in a research project should be capable of making the decision to participate and of expressing his or her preferences. Decisional capacity has been described as having several components: the physical and cognitive ability to communicate effectively; the intellectual ability to take in new information and understand, work with, and apply ("rationally manipulate") it; and the integrated cognitive and emotional ability to make sense of the meaning and repercussions of the decision within the context of one's life ("appreciation"). Interventions to help support an individual's decisional capacity may include treatment for impairing symptoms; careful and open discussions with research staff; inclusion in the consent process of family members, spouses, and "significant others" whom the participant wishes to be present; and conversations with other research participants.

Voluntarism

Authentic voluntarism or autonomy is a third necessary element of informed consent. It may be understood as involving four domains: 1) developmental factors; 2) illness-related considerations; 3) psychological issues and cultural and religious values; and 4) external features and pressures. Voluntarism is a difficult concept to operationalize, because there are so many subtle influences upon an individual's true ability to make fully independent decisions and to act freely in certain situations or at specific points in time. For example, a man whose use of substances impairs his insight and motivation may not be able to fully understand his own genuine internal wishes or to work toward enacting his own personal choices. A parent who is immensely concerned about a seriously ill child may make decisions out of desperation. Similarly, an individual who is approached by his or her teacher, employer, nursing home director, longtime personal physician, military superior, or prison warden to participate in research may not feel able to refuse. A poor person may have such need for the financial compensation associated with a study that the level of risk seems irrelevant. Finally, an elderly, ethnic minority person without health insurance may feel that he or she has few options when interacting with a clinical investigator who offers health care as part of a protocol "package." Under most circumstances, the criterion of "voluntarism" is superficially fulfilled by the absence of overt coercive influences (Roberts 2002). However, such problems associated with autonomy provide further reason for the absolute integrity of investigators as a precondition for ethical human research.

The activities surrounding informed consent thus should be designed to support information disclosure, to enhance the participant's decisional abilities, and to promote individual autonomy. The consent form represents only one concrete but important portion of the consent procedure. As such, the consent form should be clear and readable, contain relevant information, and clarify the voluntary nature of the participant's enrollment in the experiment.

Clinical observation and empirical studies indicate that there are a number of issues that bear careful consideration in informed consent for participation in psychiatric investigation. First, several studies suggest that people with psychiatric illnesses, when compared with non–psychiatrically ill control subjects or medically ill individuals, have greater difficulty taking in, retaining, and recalling information presented at the time of consent disclosures for clinical care and research procedures. The 1995 MacArthur Treatment Competence Study explored these *cognitive elements* inherent to clinical consent in 498 individuals from three groups: patients with schizophrenia or major depression, patients with ischemic heart disease, and nonpatient community volunteers. When acutely ill, the psychiatric patients in this work had significantly greater difficulty with decision making based on cognitive measures than did the patients with heart disease and the community volunteers (Appelbaum and Grisso 1995). Similar findings, not unexpectedly, have been documented among people with dementia as well. Second, elements beyond cognitive factors also may greatly influence consent activities and may adversely affect the decision-making capabilities of psychiatric patients—even those who appear cognitively "intact." For example, psychological distress; compromised insight; difficulties with interpersonal trust and communication; inaccurate beliefs; problems with motivation, initiative, and behavior; and relative powerlessness due to institutionalization or very severe symptomatology may all interfere with psychiatric patients' abilities to engage fully in a consent process.

Advance, Alternative, and Collaborative Decision Making

Psychiatric research, like other areas of biomedical experimentation, at times may involve individuals with fluctuating or declining decisional abilities. For this reason, the primary ethical safeguard for human research, informed consent, may pose special problems in psychiatric experimentation. Advance, alternative or surrogate, and collaborative decision making therefore play a particularly important role in psychiatric research consent.

Advance decision making involves careful anticipatory planning by investigators with their study participants to examine situations that may arise in the course of experimentation and to clarify the participant's own preferences in each possible situation. This process should be carefully documented ("the psychiatric advance directive") and can be enormously helpful if the participant becomes decisionally compromised or incapable. An alternative or surrogate decision maker may be designated by the participant as well to help with the implementation of the documented advance directives. Sometimes alternative decision makers may be identified or formally appointed in the absence of documented preferences of the participant, or unexpected issues arise that were not identified in advance. In these contexts, it is critical that the decision makers seek to determine or perhaps "extrapolate" what the preferences of the participant *would be,* and to make decisions accordingly. In other words, the alternative or surrogate decision maker's task is to act faithfully and to adhere closely, to whatever extent possible, to the wishes of the individual participant. Collecting data on the participant's life values (see Appendix B: The Values History in Chapter 11) and past decisions, either directly from the individual or from family members, may facilitate this process. Only when the patient's own preferences are unknowable should a "best interests" standard for substitute decision making be employed.

All forms of decision making in the context of research participation should be viewed as collaborative in nature. A collaboration takes place between participant and investigator, and in these difficult circumstances of decisional impairment, decision making may ultimately be shared by participants, spouses, family members, significant others, pastors or other individuals important to the participant, and members of the larger research team. This collaboration can be unwieldy, and confidentiality boundaries should be clarified in advance whenever possible in order to safeguard the participant's personal information. However, such collaborative efforts also help to build trust, to address problems and poor outcomes constructively, and to protect participants.

Additional Expert and Peer Review Processes

Additional expert and peer review processes may occur formally or informally. Within institutions, additional reviews may occur when seeking funding, space, or other resources or when requesting permission to perform research in certain settings. Recent guidelines for research involving special populations have suggested that protocol review be undertaken on a scale larger than individual institutions. In a highly controversial step, the National Bioethics Advisory Commission report of December 1998 recommended the development of a national review panel for all proposed research that poses greater than minimal risk to participants who have limited decision-making abilities (National Bioethics Advisory Commission 1998). Protocols may also undergo additional review and systematic monitoring through data and safety monitoring boards (DSMBs) to help ensure the safety of participants. Whereas IRBs were widely adopted in the late 1970s, DSMBs have only recently been introduced for safeguarding participants in clinical trials. They serve to evaluate trial procedures and data as they are gathered to determine whether participants are being exposed to inordinate or unexpected risks. Protections also exist after data have been gathered and analyzed. When manuscripts are submitted for publication or scientific presentations are given, the scientific and, more recently, the ethical rigor of the study often receives careful scrutiny. Because they allow for both prospective and retrospective evaluation and incorporate precise expert attention, these additional review activities are likely to become increasingly important in the repertoire of ethical safeguards.

Confidentiality Protections

Confidentiality is a privilege accorded to patients and to research participants that derives from the legal right of privacy and the ethical principle of respect for persons. In essence, the personal material gathered from and discovered about a research participant must be kept safe in all stages of data collection, analysis, and disclosure (e.g., publication, presentation). In many cases, this will mean that data will be confidentially recorded and encoded and perhaps analyzed in aggregate for scientific presentations and publications. Data should not be traceable to specific individuals unless this is specially consented to, as is the case in videotaped personal interviews of participants. Posthumous publication of personal narratives, similarly, is ethically very problematic unless special efforts to obtain consent from the individual in advance—or, perhaps, from family members or advocates who act in accordance with the values and "best interests" of the individual—are undertaken.

■ EXPERTISE, INTEGRITY, AND CONFLICTS OF INTEREST

Scientific *expertise* is critical to the ethical conduct of research. This idea is based on the notion that investigators should be knowledgeable and scientifically astute in order to ever justify the inclusion of human beings in an experiment as "a means to an end"—

namely, the pursuit of scientific findings. In established areas of science, potential investigators should show mastery of their field of study. In newer areas of science, or when investigators newly enter their scientific careers, it is important that additional expertise be gathered from mentors and collaborators whose insights may help to foster the scientific excellence of the work and help to prevent mistakes that may place study participants at unnecessary risk. Moreover, by wide consensus, the proposed science must itself possess some fundamental, significant good for society. Science for the sake of science is not sufficient. To learn something *solely for the purpose of knowing it,* especially when the process of learning it may involve potential risk or overt cruelty such as occurred in some past experimentation, is not acceptable within current ethical and moral standards. In practical terms, this means that the investigators must be capable of crafting a scientifically rigorous design, of conducting the experiment carefully and skillfully, and of interpreting the study's findings in a way that brings about direct benefit or greater knowledge that, in turn, may ultimately benefit others.

Scientific *integrity* is a necessary precondition for ethically sound scientific research. It is defined as the researcher's faithfulness, both in motivation and conduct, to the ethical duties associated with his or her professional role. For example, the scientist must intend—and act with—honesty in his or her dealings with participants and colleagues. It is upon integrity that trust—the foundation of the profession of medicine and the field of science—is built. Without trust, informed consent, institutional review, and all other safeguards would be meaningless.

Significant threats to investigator integrity represent *conflicts of interest,* defined as motivations or situations in which health care professionals' "responsibilities to observe, judge, and act according to the moral requirements of their role are, or will be, compromised" (Shimm and Spece 1996, p. 1). Conflicts of interest may arise, for example, when investigators receive very large monetary incentives for enrolling individual participants in protocols or when investigators have large financial investment in the research enterprise itself or the pharmaceutical company sponsoring the protocol. Subtler, less concrete conflicts of interest may exist as well, such as the academic investigator's desire for institutional promotion and national recognition in conjunction with an experiment. Consequently, the investigator's faithfulness to his or her moral responsibilities within the clinician investigator role—that is, the capacity and commitment to serve with integrity—is important to the ethical conduct of human research.

Integrity is especially critical in human experimentation, in part because of the inherently conflicting "dual roles" of the clinician-investigator. For instance, the dual role of the clinical investigator may create conflicts when the good of the patient is subordinated to the needs of science. Arguably, this occurs every time a patient is placed on an experimental treatment or a placebo when a known effective treatment for the patient's disorder exists. The moral obligations of this dual role raise the problem of the "therapeutic misconception" with prospective study participants. This problem, simply put, is that participants may *believe* that the clinical investigator will always act to promote the well-being of the individual participant. This beneficent aim is a fundamental expectation of other relationships with medical professionals, but is not the exclusive aim of the clinical investigator who must also serve the scientific goal of the experiment (Appelbaum et al. 1982). This is perhaps most obvious in double-blind studies, in which clinical investigators themselves are not aware of the treatment received by individual study participants.

It is important to note that this potentially conflictual role of the clinical investigator does not represent an inherent conflict of interest, as has been suggested by some. However, to minimize ethical problems associated with the dual role, there should be no other elements that threaten the ability of the investigator to think and behave in accordance with the moral aspects of his or her role. The research participant should be truly aware of the dual demands faced by the clinical investigator. And, finally, the research participant should consent in an informed and autonomous manner to "collaborate" with the investigator in the experiment.

■ SPECIAL GROUPS AND POTENTIALLY VULNERABLE POPULATIONS

Vulnerability is a concept related to the ideal of what makes us fully human—that is, the capacities and freedoms that allow us to think, to love, to desire, to work, to experience, to use language, to act intentionally, to choose authentically, to nurture, to serve others, and the like. These capacities and freedoms reside within the self, integrated in the individual person through experience, self-reflection, thought, feeling, and behavior. From a theoretical perspective, the person who is truly vulnerable cannot or does not fulfill these capacities and freedoms, singly or in an integrated manner.

More concretely, special groups and potentially vulnerable populations can be conceptualized in relation to their members' potential capacities for informed consent. Individuals whose capacity for consent is more likely to be compromised because of problems with information processing, decisional abilities, capacity for effective communication, and/or other problems related to intrinsic or extrinsic susceptibility to coercion are considered to be potentially vulnerable. This is because these individuals experience heightened risk of exploitation or, at least, have diminished ability to advocate for themselves. This concept has been extended on theoretical grounds to highly diverse groups such as severely ill medical and psychiatric patients; children; women of childbearing age; very poor people; institutionalized, "captive," or dependent individuals (e.g., prisoners, nursing home residents, students, veterans); and others. The concept of vulnerability also encompasses severely developmentally disabled people who have never been decisionally capable and seriously cognitively impaired elderly persons who have lost their independent decision-making abilities. Some theorists extend the concept of vulnerability to further include human tissues deriving from fetuses, in vitro experiments, and cadavers (Advisory Committee on Human Radiation Experiments 1996).

In recent years, biomedical science and society at large have struggled with how to best protect potentially vulnerable individuals *without* being prejudicial or disrespectful of personhood, *with-*

out usurping personal autonomy, and *without* denying access to potentially beneficial or otherwise highly valuable research endeavors. Significant efforts to develop ethically rigorous, genuinely respectful, and culturally sensitive participatory research guidelines have been undertaken (Wallerstein 1999). Significant controversies have arisen in neuropsychiatric research regarding these issues, most notably in the research areas of schizophrenia, dementia, and childhood disorders. Advocates of psychiatric investigation describe the immense suffering associated with mental illnesses and the importance of their study to clinical medicine, science, and society. Those who oppose psychiatric research express concern about the adequacy of ethical safeguards and the past exploitation of this special group of individuals with multiple sources of vulnerability. Nearly all agree, however, that psychiatric research requires very special attention and safeguards to address the ethical complexities that will inevitably arise in such work (Table 16–2) (Dresser 1996).

TABLE 16–2. **Questions to consider in areas related to the ethical acceptability of psychiatric research protocols**

---

1. Scientific issues

Is the study scientifically valuable?

Are the hypotheses adequately tested?

Can the design and methods yield meaningful data?

Does the protocol employ fully justifiable scientific techniques, either traditional or innovative?

2. Research team and context issues

Does the investigative team have enough expertise and support to successfully complete the experiment?

Is the institutional context sufficient to allow the research to progress smoothly?

Are the researchers aware of research ethics issues and potential problems related to the protocol?

Are they in good standing within the scientific and professional communities?

TABLE 16–2.	**Questions to consider in areas related to the ethical acceptability of psychiatric research protocols** *(continued)*

What conflicting roles and conflicts of interest exist in relation to this protocol? How will they be dealt with?

Are the documentation features of the protocol adequate to monitor procedures and the professional accountability of the research team?

3. Design issues related to *risk*

Does the design minimize experimental risks to participants? Do alternative designs pose less risk?

Does the protocol pose excessive risk to individual participants, the community, and/or larger society?

If participants are likely to have emerging symptoms as a result of or during protocol involvement:

- Has an appropriate mechanism for identifying and following symptom progression been built into the protocol?
- Have criteria for disenrollment from the protocol been clarified?
- Has an appropriate mechanism for providing alternative or traditional treatment been established?

4. Design issues related to *benefit*

What benefits exist for participants? Are benefits and their likelihood accurately described?

Have benefits of the study been optimized for individuals and society without being coercive to potential participants?

Is it expected that societal benefit derived from the protocol be specifically applicable to the population being studied?

5. Confidentiality

Is participant information carefully safeguarded during the collection, storage, and analysis stages of the study?

6. Selection, exclusion, and recruitment issues

Does the process of selection, exclusion, and recruitment ensure that members of vulnerable populations, as they are currently defined, are included *only* if essential to the study's scientific hypotheses?

Are understudied populations inappropriately excluded from participation, i.e., are selection and recruitment practices potentially discriminatory?

Is the recruitment process itself noncoercive?

TABLE 16–2.	Questions to consider in areas related to the ethical acceptability of psychiatric research protocols *(continued)*

7. Informed consent and decisional capacity issues

Does the informed consent disclosure process include all relevant information, such as:

- the study's purpose and the nature of the illness or the phenomenon being studied
- who is responsible for the scientific and ethical conduct of the study
- why the individual may be eligible for participation
- the proposed intervention and its associated risks and benefits and their relative likelihood alternatives to participation
- key study design features (e.g., placebo use, randomization, medication-free intervals, frequency of visits, confidentiality, plans for use of data)

Is there reasonable assurance of adequate decisional capacity of participants with respect to the ability to understand, rationally analyze, and appreciate the meaning of the research decision?

If participants have or are at risk for diminished decisional capacity at any time during protocol participation:

- Have efforts for enhancing or restoring the decisional capacity of the participant been undertaken?
- Is there an appropriate mechanism for identifying, following, and documenting participants' level of diminished decisional capacity?
- Does the protocol include an appropriate mechanism for advance decision making by the participant or for identifying an alternative decision maker for the participant? Is it clear when the advance directive or alternative decision maker should be put into effect?

Is the consent form concise, readable, accurate, and understandable?

Is there reasonable assurance that individuals will not experience coercive pressure to participate in the project or continue in the project?

8. Incentive issues

Are incentives for participation sufficient and timed so that they compensate research participants *without* being coercive?

If health care is an incentive, how will the patient's health care needs be met if disenrollment becomes necessary?

TABLE 16–2. **Questions to consider in areas related to the ethical acceptability of psychiatric research protocols** *(continued)*

9. Review issues

Has the protocol undergone appropriate scientific and ethical review?

Should the protocol undergo any additional review steps (e.g., by community leaders)?

Does the protocol have features (e.g., very high risk, very vulnerable participants) that merit ongoing external monitoring?

10. Data presentation/authorship issues

Will the presentation of the data describe the ethical safeguards employed in the protocol?

Will the presentation of the data meet current ethical standards with respect to authorship?

Will the presentation of the data meet other current standards, e.g., accurate disclosure of conflicting roles and conflicts of interest?

Will participants' identities be adequately protected in data presentation?

Source. Adapted from Roberts et al. 2001.

■ ANIMAL RESEARCH

Animal research is highly controversial and can be deeply troubling, in part because the primary safeguard of informed consent allowing for authentic autonomous collaboration is not possible. In general, responsibilities to animals have been characterized as avoiding inflicting unnecessary pain, deprivation, and suffering; protecting welfare by improving the environment; searching for alternatives to the use of animals; and setting policies and performing professional review that define and uphold ethical standards within animal experimentation. The conduct of animal research is guided by the "three R's" of *replacing* animals with nonanimal research methods (e.g., computer models, experiments with tissues), *reducing* the numbers of animals in experiments, and *refining* experimental techniques to minimize harm to experimental animals. Animal research is carefully reviewed and regulated on an institutional basis. Nevertheless, problems exist, for example, with the educational uses of animals in medicine and the lack of consensus about the necessity for the very extensive use of animals in experiments prior to approval and release of medications in this country. Investigation of psychiatric phenomena employing animal models poses two special issues in comparison with other areas of medicine: the study of pathological behavior that is sometimes induced to allow for animal experimentation and the relatively frequent use of more neurologically and socially sophisticated animals such as nonhuman primates (Orlans et al. 1998).

■ PRACTICAL EFFORTS REGARDING THE ETHICAL CONDUCT OF RESEARCH

To be ethically sound, psychiatric research should remain faithful to the principles of *respect for persons, beneficence,* and *justice;* be conducted by investigators who possess expertise and integrity; have justifiable design and methods; and uphold safeguards shared throughout the field of biomedical research. A number of efforts can be made to assess and ensure the ethical conduct of research. Review of the list of questions in each of the domains provided in Table 16–2 may be helpful to prospective investigators, protocol reviewers, or concerned readers of scientific literature. In addition, the Roberts Research Protocol Ethics Assessment Tool (RePEAT), an educational tool for reviewing and writing protocols is presented in the Appendix to this chapter. Animal research poses important issues of which psychiatric investigators should remain aware. Finally, special efforts to address the attributes and circumstances of people with mental illness may further help to mitigate against, and even to reverse, their potential vulnerabilities with respect to participating in human research.

Case Scenarios

A researcher struggles with the question of whether to enroll a homeless person diagnosed with schizophrenia in a medication protocol. She is concerned that the patient will feel coerced by the free medication and health care he will receive if he enrolls and that the patient will have few resources if he becomes seriously symptomatic and demands discharge during the medication-free run-in period.

A researcher who owns stock in a major pharmaceutical company becomes a primary investigator on a trial for a new medication.

A researcher fails to report several adverse events to the institutional review board of the institution at which he is conducting research.

A junior researcher wants to test a new herbal medication in patients with panic disorder. The medication in question has undergone very few basic science studies of its safety or efficacy.

A researcher is concerned that several of the patients in his neuroimaging study of dementia are not decisionally capable. However, because the study poses minimal risks to participants, he allows them to remain in the study if they give assent and have a responsible surrogate decision maker.

■ REFERENCES

Advisory Committee on Human Radiation Experiments: The Human Radiation Experiments: Final Report of the President's Advisory Committee. New York, Oxford University Press, 1996

Appelbaum P, Grisso T: The MacArthur Competence Study I, II, III. Law and Human Behavior 19:105–174, 1995

Appelbaum PS, Roth LH, Lidz C: The therapeutic misconception: informed consent in psychiatric research. Int J Law Psychiatry 5(3–4):319–329, 1982

Dresser R: Mentally disabled research subjects. The enduring policy issues. JAMA 276:67–72, 1996

Levine RJ: Ethics and Regulation of Clinical Research. Baltimore, MD, Urban & Schwarzenberg, 1986

National Bioethics Advisory Commission: Research Involving Subjects With Mental Disorders That May Affect Decisionmaking Capacity. Rockville, MD, National Bioethics Advisory Commission, 1998

National Commission for the Protection of Human Subjects of Biomedical and Behavioral Research: The Belmont Report: Ethical Principles and Guidelines for the Protection of Human Subjects of Research. Washington, DC, U.S. Government Printing Office, 1979

Orlans FB, Beauchamp TL, Dresser R, et al: The Human Use of Animals: Case Studies in Ethical Choice. Oxford, UK, Oxford University Press, 1998

Roberts LW: The ethical basis of psychiatric research: conceptual issues and empirical findings. Compr Psychiatry 39:99–110, 1998

Roberts LW: Informed consent and the capacity for voluntarism. Am J Psychiatry 159:705–712, 2002

Roberts LW, Geppert CMA, Brody JL: A framework for considering the ethical aspects of psychiatric research protocols. Compr Psychiatry 42:351–363, 2001

Shimm DS, Spece RG Jr: Introduction, in Conflicts of Interest in Clinical Practice and Research. Edited by Spece RG Jr, Shimm DS, Buchanan AE. New York, Oxford University Press, 1996, pp 1–11

Wallerstein N: Power between evaluator and community: research relationships within New Mexico's healthier communities. Soc Sci Med 49:39–53, 1999

Appendix

ROBERTS RESEARCH PROTOCOL ETHICS ASSESSMENT TOOL (RePEAT)

APPENDIX. Roberts Research Protocol Ethics Assessment Tool (RePEAT)	Acceptable		Unacceptable	
Scientific merit and design issues				
1. Do the study's hypotheses possess *scientific merit?*	Yes	Not applicable	Requires clarification	No
2. Does the *research design appropriately test* its hypotheses?	Yes	Not applicable	Requires clarification	No
Expertise, commitment, and integrity issues				
3. Does the research team have sufficient *expertise* to successfully conduct the study?	Yes	Not applicable	Requires clarification	No
4. Does the research team have sufficient *commitment, resources, and support* from the institution to successfully conduct the study?	Yes	Not applicable	Requires clarification	No
5. Are the members of the research team *knowledgeable* with respect to the ethics of human research and in *good standing* within the scientific and professional communities?	Yes	Not applicable	Requires clarification	No
6. Does evidence exist of *past misconduct* by members of the research team, individually or collectively?	No	No	Requires clarification	Yes
7. Do the financial, institutional, or other arrangements related to the protocol pose any *threat to the integrity* of members of the research team, individually or collectively (e.g., significant "conflicts of interest")?	No	No	Requires clarification	Yes

APPENDIX. Roberts Research Protocol Ethics Assessment Tool (RePEAT) (continued)

	Acceptable		Unacceptable	
Risks and benefits				
8. Are *experimental risks* to participants minimized by the research design?	Yes	Not applicable	Requires clarification	No
9. Does the protocol pose *excessive risk or other burdens* to individual participants, the community, and/or larger society?	No	Not applicable	Requires clarification	Yes
10. If participants are likely to have *emerging symptoms* (i.e., appearance of new symptoms or worsening of existing symptoms) as a result of or during protocol participation:				
a. has an appropriate mechanism for *identifying and following symptom progression* been built into the protocol?	Yes	Not applicable	Requires clarification	No
b. has an appropriate mechanism for *identifying when to discontinue protocol participation* in order to begin standard treatment for emerging symptoms that pose safety risks or involve enduring distress been built into the protocol?	Yes	Not applicable	Requires clarification	No
c. has an appropriate mechanism for *referring or providing patients with standard treatment* for emerging symptoms that pose safety risks or enduring distress been built into protocol?	Yes	Not applicable	Requires clarification	No

APPENDIX. Roberts Research Protocol Ethics Assessment Tool (RePEAT) *(continued)*

		Acceptable	Unacceptable	
11. Are *benefits* in association with research participation optimized by the research design for individuals and society?	Yes	Not applicable	Requires clarification	No
Confidentiality				
12. Do the research design and plans for data use adequately protect participant *confidentiality?*	Yes	Not applicable	Requires clarification	No
Participant selection and recruitment				
13. Does the selection and recruitment process for the protocol ensure that members of *vulnerable populations* (e.g., children, institutionalized or decisionally impaired patients, women who are pregnant or may become pregnant) will be included only if essential to the study's scientific hypotheses?	Yes	Not applicable	Requires clarification	No
14. Are *understudied populations* inappropriately excluded from participation, i.e., are selection and recruitment practices potentially discriminatory?	No	Not applicable	Requires clarification	Yes
15. Does the *selection and recruitment process* for the protocol ensure that potential participants may comfortably refuse protocol involvement, i.e., is the recruitment process itself noncoercive?	Yes	Not applicable	Requires clarification	No

APPENDIX. Roberts Research Protocol Ethics Assessment Tool (RePEAT) *(continued)*		Acceptable	Unacceptable	
16. Will benefits derived from the protocol, if any, be conferred to the specific *population being studied* in the protocol?	Yes	Not applicable	Requires clarification	No
Informed consent and decisional capacity				
17. Does the research design define an appropriate *informed consent process* including:				
a. *disclosure of information* regarding: —the study's purpose —who is responsible for the conduct of the study —why the individual may be eligible for participation —the nature of the illness (or the phenomenon being studied) —the proposed intervention —the associated risks and benefits and their relative likelihood —alternatives to participation —key study design features (e.g., placebo use, randomization, medication-free intervals, frequency of visits, confidentiality, plans for use of data) and other issues?	Yes	Not applicable	Requires clarification	No

APPENDIX.	Roberts Research Protocol Ethics Assessment Tool (RePEAT) *(continued)*		
	Acceptable	Unacceptable	No
b. reasonable assurance of adequate *decisional capacity* of participants with respect to the ability to understand, rationally analyze, and appreciate the meaning of the research decision, OR reasonable assurance of adequately meeting all criteria listed under Item 18 below?	Yes	Not applicable	Requires clarification	No
c. reasonable assurance that individuals will *not experience coercive pressure* to participate during the consent phase or during protocol involvement (e.g., timing of consent discussions so that individuals can think through the decision and seek advice from others; explicit acknowledgement that participation is voluntary and that individuals may refuse or withdraw from protocol involvement without adverse consequences; giving even decisionally incapable participants the right to refuse)?	Yes	Not applicable	Requires clarification	No
d. a *concise, readable, accurate, and understandable* consent form, suited to the population under study?	Yes	Not applicable	Requires clarification	No

APPENDIX.	Roberts Research Protocol Ethics Assessment Tool (RePEAT) *(continued)*		
		Acceptable	Unacceptable
18. If participants are likely to experience *diminished decisional capacity at any time* during protocol participation (including at the time of enrollment):			
a. has an appropriate mechanism for *identifying, following, and documenting the level of diminished decisional capacity* of participants been built into the protocol?	Yes	Not applicable	Requires clarification	No
b. when possible, has an appropriate mechanism for *enhancing or restoring the decisional capacity* of the participant been built into the protocol?	Yes	Not applicable	Requires clarification	No
c. if a *period of diminished decisional capacity may be necessary* because of the scientific hypotheses of the study (e.g., a study of advanced dementia or of some life-threatening emergencies, or a psychopharmacology trial study involving a relatively brief medication-free interval), does the protocol include:			
1) an appropriate mechanism for *advance decision making by the participant or for identifying an alternative decision maker* for the participant?	Yes	Not applicable	Requires clarification	No
2) an appropriate mechanism for *implementing advance decisions or for preparing and utilizing the alternative decision maker* when necessary?	Yes	Not applicable	Requires clarification	No

APPENDIX. Roberts Research Protocol Ethics Assessment Tool (RePEAT) *(continued)*			

Incentives

19. Are *incentives for participation* sufficient and appropriately timed so that they compensate research participants *without* being coercive? — Yes / Not applicable / Requires clarification / No

Other issues

20. Are the *documentation* practices adequate to monitor protocol procedures and the professional accountability of the research team? — Yes / Not applicable / Requires clarification / No

21. Is an appropriate "debriefing" process built into the protocol so that participants may be informed of relevant study procedures and/or findings? — Yes / Not applicable / Requires clarification / No

22. Are *other ethical problems* apparent in this protocol?
If "yes," describe: — No / Not applicable / Requires clarification / Yes

23. Are there *other issues that interfere with protocol approval?*
If "yes," describe: — No / Not applicable / Requires clarification / Yes

24. Prior to its approval, does the protocol require *additional review* by others with more specialized expertise or by others with especially relevant interests and experience to assess its ethics or its science? — No / Not applicable / Requires clarification / Yes

APPENDIX.	Roberts Research Protocol Ethics Assessment Tool (RePEAT) *(continued)*		
Does the protocol, *in its present form*, meet minimal criteria for being ethically sound?*		Yes	No
Does the protocol, *in its present form*, require a more rigorous level of monitoring than is customary?		Yes	No
Comment:			

Note. This tool is intended for use in assessment of ethical aspects of research protocols involving human participants.

*All evaluative criteria (Items 1–24) must receive an acceptable response for the protocol to be *minimally acceptable* on ethical grounds. Problems, as indicated by responses in *either* of the second two columns, should be addressed formally and should undergo re-review prior to protocol approval.

Source. Copyright 1999, Laura Weiss Roberts, M.D.

17

HEALTH CARE
ETHICS COMMITTEES

With Tom Townsend, M.D.

Whereas the responsibility for ethical decision making often resides within the individual, the professions also have a responsibility to their members and to society to oversee the activities that are entrusted to them. Individual knowledge, skill, and conscience are not enough. Furthermore, there may be legitimate differences in values, preferences, and judgments between patient and clinician, between family and patient, and among health care professionals. Some social and administrative mechanism is needed, short of judicial review, to air, clarify, and find common ground among these differences so that actions may be taken in caring for patients. Health care ethics committees represent one approach to this need; in this chapter, we review the development of such committees and their application to clinical practice.

■ THE RISE OF HEALTH CARE
ETHICS COMMITTEES

It is helpful to review some of reasons for the claim that decisions by committees in hospitals have moral significance. Whereas the modern bioethics movement has its origins in the 1960s, the last half of the twentieth century saw the recognition and buttressing of global civil rights—not just the rights to guarantee racial fairness, but the rights of all groups at risk: children, women, those with mental illness or handicaps, and, almost by definition (*patient* means suffering), the medically ill. These individual rights were developing at the same time that modern medicine was developing technologies to prolong life and reduce suffering. These interventions changed practice in the care of premature newborns in the neonatal intensive care unit, of permanently unconscious patients, and of patients with advanced renal failure. Concurrently, controversies related to dubious research practices, definitions of legal and clinical death, abortion rights and legislation, and new strains on access to health care arose (Ross 1986; Ross et al. 1993). Responses to these events led to a new mechanism for critical thinking about making difficult, ethically laden choices—in this case, decision by committee.

■ HISTORICAL BACKGROUND: SOME NOTABLE FAULTY MEDICAL RESEARCH PRACTICES

The most direct antecedent of the hospital ethics committee was the institutional review board (IRB), which arose out of the national response to reports of abuses of human subjects in research in which moral claims for informed consent were severely breached (see Chapter 16). Many examples of such abuses were listed by Beecher (1966) in his landmark article "Ethics and Clinical Research." Of special concern was that these research disasters in the United States occurred in the aftermath of the 1946 Nuremberg Trials of Nazi physicians, where it was revealed that involuntary "research" had been done on human beings, resulting in tremendous suffering and even death. The worldwide outrage in response to this discovery led to development of the Nuremberg Code of Ethics, which contained 10 requirements for dealing with the ethics of experimentation on human participants (Katz 1996). This code of ethics was intended to recognize and to guarantee the rights of each subject as an individual, as well as protect the subjects' welfare. Regrettably, that rather plain and unassailable goal was not to be achieved in the United States for several years.

To illustrate, we will consider three examples. In 1963, elderly patients with chronic illnesses living at the Jewish Chronic Disease Hospital in Brooklyn were injected with live cancer cells to see if the cells would survive in ill patients without cancer. Although the researchers apparently did not believe that the cells would remain viable, or induce cancer, they did the experiment without any fore-warning and without bothering to obtain consent from either patients or their family. In 1932, the U.S. Public Health Service began research on African American men in impoverished rural Tuskegee, Alabama, to discover the natural course of tertiary syphilis. Patients were followed closely with examinations and blood tests, but were provided no therapy, even after penicillin became available in the 1940s. Some invasive tests (e.g., lumbar punctures to study spinal fluid) were even presented as therapy. The study continued until reported to the public in a newspaper article in 1972. That article prompted a review by the U.S. Department of Health, Education, and Welfare (DHEW), which concluded that the study had been "ethically unjustified" from its inception. Finally, in 1967, it was discovered that ongoing research at the Willowbrook State School in New York had been exposing mentally retarded institutionalized children to hepatitis to observe the course of the disease. Although this "research" occurred at a time when the disease was not well understood and a vaccine was not yet available—and during an era when many institutionalized individuals contracted hepatitis, it emerged that the institution's admission policy accorded preference to children whose families had "volunteered" them for the research (Fletcher et al. 1997).

Once revealed, these and other research debacles prompted Congress to create the National Commission for the Protection of Human Subjects of Biomedical and Behavioral Research in 1974. The commission subsequently developed *The Belmont Report: Ethical Principles and Guidelines for the Protection of Human Subjects of Research* (National Commission for the Protection of Human Subjects of Biomedical and Behavioral Research 1979). From the Commission's work, and the *Belmont Report,* came a recommendation that any research involving human subjects be reviewed locally by IRBs. IRBs were to include not only researchers but also, importantly, lay members to contribute vital community perspectives that might otherwise be overlooked. This important addition to committee membership modeled the way that hospital ethics committees would be constituted (Fletcher et al. 1997; Ross 1986).

■ EARLY FORMS OF HOSPITAL ETHICS COMMITTEES

Compelling patient care issues that propelled the development of health care ethics committees in the 1960s and 1970s often involved moral dilemmas created by the difficult decisions of how to best use developing technologies. For instance, hemodialysis for chronic renal disease was developed in the 1930s by Willem Kolff and was used after the war, but there was not a technology that allowed repeated use until Belding Scribner, a physician in Seattle, made an artery-to-vein shunt that could be reused. Scribner's first patient, Clyde Shields, lived 11 years after Scribner's discovery. Although the new technology represented an astonishing advance for individuals previously doomed to uremia, or renal toxicity, and death, it initially was available only in Seattle. This meant that despite the immediate demand for the machines, there was only limited access. In fact, a patient had to live in Washington State to receive dialysis in the hospital where Scribner worked, the University of Washington.

To guide the decision of rationing use of these scarce and expensive "artificial kidney machines," the hospital recruited an anonymous committee of lay members from the community to review candidates and offer the procedure or not, depending on the committee's judgment about the relative social worth of the individuals. The committee, colloquially known as "the God Committee," became notorious after an article describing its deliberations appeared in *Life* magazine (Alexander 1962). Although the article was favorable toward dialysis, the committee's role led to considerable controversy and increased media attention to medical ethics issues in general.

We are continually reminded of the significance of the potential to prolong life with dialysis, and the committee's way of dealing with it, in the development of the field of bioethics. In 2002, Kolff and Scribner (91 and 81 years old, respectively, at the time) received the Lasker Award for Medical Research for their work with the early dialysis units. The award citation stated that dialysis not only transformed kidney failure from a fatal disease to a treatable one but also spawned the discipline of medical ethics (Altman 2002).

Not too much later, in 1967, organ transplantation with a human heart was successfully performed in South Africa by Christiaan Barnard. This event signaled substantial changes in medicine and health care ethics attitudes. Its significance for institutional ethics committees became clear within a year, when the Harvard Medical School's Ad Hoc Committee to Examine the Definition of Brain Death (1968) published its findings. The committee had worked to establish the criteria that would be used to pronounce death in patients being kept on respirators until their organs could be retrieved for transplantation. Subsequent legislation derived from the President's Commission included a Uniform Determination of Death Act. Thus, the very difficult issues of determining who should receive organ transplantation and delineating death were successfully addressed by an ethics committee. This committee was entrusted with acting responsibly within a health care institution to influence national policy without waiting for persons or organizations outside medicine to develop such policies.

In 1976, the New Jersey Supreme Court heard the case of Karen Ann Quinlan, a young woman in a coma who was requiring ventilator support to live. The significance of this landmark case for bioethics was immense. In their decision, judges at the Supreme Court level had clearly been impressed by a current article (Teel 1975) stating that "many hospitals have established an ethics committee…which serves to review the individual circumstances of ethics dilemmas…" and act in an advisory capacity to the clinical team. The justices, in their decision on whether to allow disconnection of the respirator at the request of the family, ruled that if Quinlan's attending physician determined that there was no reasonable chance that she would ever return to a "cognitive, sapient state," and if the hospital ethics committee (they called it a "prognosis committee") agreed with that prognosis, then the family's request for withdrawal could be granted. The Court decision suggested to the medical community that end-of-life health care issues needed to stay out of the judicial system when possible.

In 1983, the President's Commission for the Study of Ethical Problems in Medicine and Biomedical and Biobehavioral Research published "Deciding to Forgo Life-Sustaining Treatment." The commission recognized that the many difficult treatment decisions surrounding life-prolonging therapies offered to adults with compromised decisional capacity and seriously ill newborns would require committees to protect the interests of incapacitated patients in the decisions to forgo life-sustaining treatment. They understood that these ethics committees could not fully safeguard patients against potential harm, but they believed that attempts to educate, recommend policy, and review cases would increase the likelihood that these tough decisions would be made locally and without repeated forays into court; in fact, the commission hoped to see the courts used only as a last resort.

■ WHERE ARE ETHICS COMMITTEES TODAY?

Most professional practice organizations call for health care institutions to have some sort of ethics program, or a functional equivalent. Very importantly, since 1991, the Joint Commission for Accreditation of Healthcare Organizations (JCAHO), which sets standards and regulates the health care industry, has required a "mechanism" for the consideration of ethical issues arising in the care of patients. This mechanism, most commonly a patient care ethics committee, must also provide education to caregivers and patients on ethical issues in health care. The JCAHO dictum has now been changed to require a "functioning process to address ethical issues" in patient rights and organizational ethics. This broader language permits diverse forms of ethics activities to fulfill institutional ethics requirements.

■ WHAT DO HEALTH CARE ETHICS COMMITTEES DO?

Ethics committees have been a part of the decision-making landscape in U.S. health care since the late 1970s. But what is expected of such committees, and how would we know whether they are doing a good job? Health care ethics committees are customarily expected to play three important roles in the institution as well as the community it serves—education, policy development and review, and case consultation. Health care ethics committees perform the following activities:

- Host educational programs on salient medical ethics topics
- Create a venue for discussion of biomedical–ethical issues in the institution
- Provide advice and resources in relation to patient care decision making
- Conduct reviews of ethically important cases or decisions
- Offer guidance on institutional policies related to bioethical issues

Within an institution, the committee (or program) serves both to educate and to advise, which makes it imperative that the ethics program be available and visible. An overview of these functions follows.

Ethics Education

The educational component is essential to any ethics program, regardless of the institution's size. Education on issues of ethics and health care law should be continuously offered to health care professionals, staff, and the lay community. Ethics education in the form of ethics rounds in hospitals, particularly in intensive care units, has been shown to have a beneficial effect. In some situations these educational activities can function proactively to obviate the need for a full ethics consultation.

Educational services led by the ethics committee may serve to further educate committee members—a form of "on the job" training. It is also useful to have new ethics committee members join the committee at the same time. This shared transition period offers a kind of orientation phase in which knowledge about the history and theory of bioethics may be imparted. In addition, new members can become comfortable engaging in honest—and occasionally quite candid—moral discourse with others on the committee. Acquiring and practicing ethics skills may be enhanced by reviewing current cases, studying landmark or paradigmatic cases in the literature, role playing of important cases, and participating in general discussions of applied ethical theory. It is not difficult to engage staff or laypersons in the compelling topics of clinical and research ethics that daily headline the newspapers.

Programs just getting started usually do well to have some form of organized reading program, recruiting motivated members to lead conversations about specific issues they have identified, as well as outside regional resources and networks (including recently developed web sites). Reviewing in greater depth the general history of ethics committees outlined briefly here, and especially the various volumes of the President's Commission, are appropriate beginnings. Several in-depth introductory texts offer more support to interested learners who have had limited exposure to the literature of bioethics. Although the case-based consultations provided by ethics committees are often their most visible activities, it is the educational service of ethics committees that represents their greatest contribution to institutions.

Policy Formulation and Review

Ethics committees offer pivotal support in developing institutional policy. Although many committee members think of policy development as dull and mundane (as well as difficult and even painful, given that policies often require a year or more from drafting to implementation), such policies are critically important: by outlining what the institution says it will do, and specifying who is responsible for having it done, they offer accountability in the institution's care of patients. Examples of policies required by the JCAHO that need the consultation (or origination) of the ethics committee include informed consent, advance directives, pain management, confidentiality, treatment refusal, and Jehovah's Witnesses. The committee can serve as a forum for—or orchestrate—the necessary debate on the understanding and wording of the policy. This process nearly always involves creating differing and alternative policies and selecting the best policy for the institution after involving leaders in the institution and community. Institutional culture evolves with the appearance of new therapies and clinicians; the ethics committee and its policies act as an institutional memory and ensure that institutional policies both make sense and reflect the current culture of the institution. Also, policy development, which can be conducted effectively in subcommittee assignments, can offer a tremendous opportunity for education.

Case Consultation

Health care ethics committees may help clinicians, patients, and their families make difficult moral, as well as clinical, decisions. Ethics consultation is what many ethics committee members consider to be their core task; they are being trained to help people make ethically correct and defensible clinical decisions within the institution. As shown in Figure 17–1, developing ethical clinical practices requires the conjunction of several elements. Health care ethics committees can help apply these basic elements as they assist clinicians, patients, and families. Although ethics committees are designed to be pragmatic and thus useful to the institutions they serve, ethics case consultations are nonetheless a relatively new phenomenon. As such, their results remain rather variable, and they are not always appreciated—or even sought or permitted—by patients, families, or the health care team. As with other forms of clinical consultation, members of an ethics committee will ideally approach ethics consul-

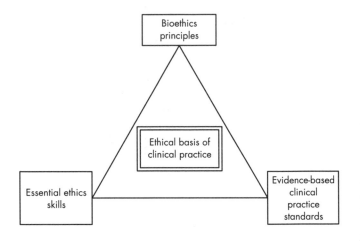

FIGURE 17–1. **The ethical basis of clinical practice: applying principles, skills, and evidence.**

tation with respect for the complexity of the patient care situation, offering assistance and expert knowledge whenever possible.

Discussion of cases is an ongoing educational goal and responsibility of ethics committees. These cases need to be explored in depth, and attempts to condense the reasoning loop (e.g., dismissing an issue of patient refusal of clearly beneficial treatment as "autonomy") may preclude appropriate assessment of the issues involved. Understanding of novel ethics issues will require that individual members of multiple disciplines and backgrounds express the variety of values they each are depended on to contribute. Committees whose members have worked together for some time and have encountered many kinds of patient care dilemmas together can often slice immediately to the core of a case. But when members are less experienced and still learning, even simple cases require complex moral discussions that go beyond mere resolution of the case. Paradigm cases, cases from workbooks or case-study books, and foundation legal cases—as well as standard texts—all provide opportunities for exploring an ethical issue.

Arriving at a clear consensus is challenging and is not always the aim of an ethics consultation. Instead, identifying solutions that are acceptable—and defining solutions that are *not* acceptable—may be a more appropriate goal.

Ethics consultations are often called simply to shed light on ethical issues commonly witnessed in the institution, without necessarily referring to a particular case. For instance, a house officer unfamiliar with the health care law about advance directives might request assistance, which will not require a full consultation; or a staff member might ask to initiate a discussion about a specific case or type of issue (e.g., a patient refusing what is deemed beneficial therapy by the health care team). These types of cases are legitimately handled without the full consultation team or the committee (Fletcher et al. 1997). Indeed, consultations may occur through an ethics committee, a subset of that committee, or an individual consultant or consultation team.

It is critical that there be institutional support for the committee and its consultation service, because consultation is a complex task with repercussions, some of which are potentially harmful. A consultation service should be careful not to take on more than it can handle—that is, the complexity of the role should correspond to the level of sophistication of the service and the resources it has available. For this reason, some services may offer only information and education, others may provide a forum for discussion but not advice, still others might serve a mediation role, and some might even handle administrative or organizational ethics issues (Fletcher et al. 1997).

Institutional policies should be explicit about how the consultation service is to be approached, who can request a consultation, the consultation service's role, what types of cases can be dealt with, whether recommendations will be offered, and when, if ever, such recommendations may be binding rather than advisory. Given the moral complexities in clinical care, most people feel that ethics consultations should be advisory only. There is always a possibility that any binding recommendation from the ethics committee will be perceived as a unilateral decision by the health care team (particularly physicians) that either does not understand—or worse, tolerate—the particular moral positioning of the patient or surrogate.

At most institutions, ethics committees may be approached for assistance by any "stakeholder" involved in a case, ranging from patient or family member to physician or hospital administrator. Nevertheless, if an ethics consultation is to be done, it is essential to notify the attending physician, regardless of whether that physician requested the consultation. It is just as important to notify and obtain the consent of the patient or surrogate, if possible.

Figure 17–2 provides a model for ethical decision making. Table 17–1 lists questions that may assist ethics discussions.

A recently published task force report from the American Society for Bioethics and the Humanities (Aulisio et al. 2000) established standards for bioethics consultation, including the nine general conclusions summarized in Table 17–2. As described earlier, there is variability in the ethics consultation process, as well as inconsistency in results in different hospital settings, or even the same hospital on different occasions. This report is particularly helpful in that it illustrates and validates the existence of these variations among responsible committees as they facilitate ethics discussions in their respective communities. The task force report emphasizes "core competencies." Importantly, the report rejects the certification of individuals and the accreditation of programs at this point in American medicine. It further affirms that building a culture of ethics sensitivity, receptiveness, knowledge, and skill represents the most important benefit of an ethics committee's efforts overall.

■ WHO SHOULD BE ON A HEALTH CARE ETHICS COMMITTEE?

Ethics conversations require the representation of divergent viewpoints in order to be comprehensive and attuned to the complexity and diversity of situations encountered in health care. Many have recognized the important role of the mental health professional in

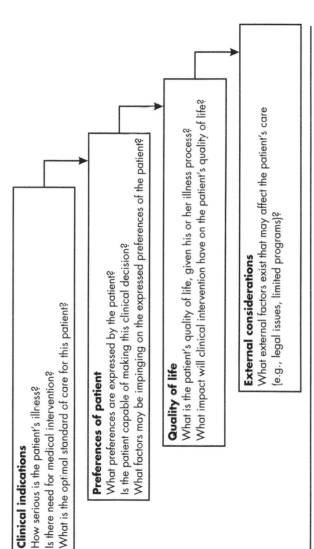

Clinical indications
How serious is the patient's illness?
Is there need for medical intervention?
What is the optimal standard of care for this patient?

Preferences of patient
What preferences are expressed by the patient?
Is the patient capable of making this clinical decision?
What factors may be impinging on the expressed preferences of the patient?

Quality of life
What is the patient's quality of life, given his or her illness process?
What impact will clinical intervention have on the patient's quality of life?

External considerations
What external factors exist that may affect the patient's care
(e.g., legal issues, limited programs)?

FIGURE 17–2. **A model for clinical ethical decision making.**

TABLE 17–1. **Questions to help guide ethics committee discussions**

1. What are the central medical considerations of this case?
2. What is the accepted standard of care for the patient? If not known, what are two or three possible courses of action that would meet current standards in this case?
3. What are the patient's preferences in this situation?
4. What is the patient's decision-making capacity? If the patient lacks capacity, what is understood about the patient's lifelong values? Are there advance directives? Is there an appropriate decision maker?
5. What are the significant human factors of the case? (Examples include patient's age, attitudes, occupation, religious beliefs, and values.)
6. Identify all of the related major value factors present for the patient, for the health care professionals, and for other relevant persons who are involved in the case. Which of these are health care values (e.g., comfort, benefit) and which are other kinds of considerations (e.g., economic, political)?
7. Identify and describe the major value conflict in the case.
8. Prioritize the ethical values that are in conflict in the case.
9. Has everyone who should be involved in the process been included?

TABLE 17–2. **Ethics consultation: conclusions of the Task Force on Standards for Bioethics Consultation**

1. U.S. societal context makes "ethics facilitation" an appropriate approach to ethics consultation.
2. Ethics facilitation requires certain core competencies.
3. Core competencies can be acquired in various ways.
4. Individual consultants, teams, or committees should have the core competencies for ethics consultation.
5. Consultation services should have policies that address access, patient notification, documentation, and case review.
6. Abuse of power and conflicts of interest must be avoided.
7. Ethics consultation must have institutional support.
8. Evaluation of process, outcomes, and competencies is needed.
9. Certification of individuals and accreditation of programs are rejected.

Source.   Adapted from Aulisio et al. 2000.

these discussions, both to provide insight into key elements of the case and to track and facilitate the committee's process of reflection and deliberation. Toleration of and receptivity to divergent viewpoints, important for cultural diversity and understanding, can also serve to win the trust of various constituencies.

Ethics committees need to include members from multiple disciplines, diverse cultures, and different walks of life. It is helpful to have a professional ethicist on the committee. Attorneys likewise can provide a valuable perspective; however, participation of the lawyer representing the hospital would constitute a conflict of interest that should be disclosed and well understood among the committee members.

Psychiatrists, psychologists, and other professionals with mental health expertise play a critically important role in health care ethics committees. Attunement to the complexities of group process and collaborative decision making combined with sophisticated knowledge of patient decisional capacity issues may facilitate optimal committee processes. Moreover, ethics consultations may be precipitated by poorly recognized psychiatric issues that exist in the case.

Finally, the personal qualities of committee members matter greatly. Committee members must possess integrity. They need to be interested in the work of the committee and the institution. They need to be respected, but that does not mean they need to be powerful. They need to be easy to talk with, willing to listen, and open to learning. They must have backbone (versus merely being oppositional), and they must be communicative (not merely talkative). A health care ethics committee is known for its ability to shape ethical behavior in the institution and the community. Influence of committee members is always dependent on the respect they have earned among colleagues, and seldom on any special skills they possess in a particular pedagogy.

■ PROFESSIONAL ASSOCIATION ETHICS COMMITTEES

Various professional organizations maintain ethics committees to review complaints from patients or clients, to educate their members on matters of ethics, and to sanction or discipline unethical members. Notably, those professions that engage in psychotherapeutic practices take these responsibilities particularly seriously. The American Psychiatric Association, the American Psychological Association, and the National Association of Social Workers maintain active ethics committees at both national and local levels. These associations have written codes of ethics or statements of ethics principles by which members agree to abide and against which complaints of unethical behavior may be judged. Professional codes and standards pertaining to ethical conduct serve both to delineate the profession's responsibility to the public and to offer guidance to its practitioners.

■ SUMMARY

More than personal morality is involved in clinical ethics. The health care profession both requires and relies on a larger practicing code, an ethos for all practitioners that defines their social role and represents the integrity of the profession. When health care practitioners breach these standards, they jeopardize not only their personal identity but also any moral presence and contribution that the profession as a whole might have in society. Professionalism is neither fully formulated nor static; rather, it is constantly evolving as reflective clinicians and outside observers call for improvements or alterations in the practice of medicine to meet changing conditions. The many advances in technological capabilities in the past few decades have been accompanied by the appearance of new and dangerous diseases, economic and insurance instability, and increasing complexity in the delivery and receipt of health care. Patients actually still regularly trust their caregivers to do, or to advocate, what is understood to be clinically and socially best for the patient. At times, however, satisfactory clinical and ethical outcomes will naturally entail the inclusion of consultation with a committee specially constituted to help deliberate over choices and to represent diverse and complex views in the service of the patient's interests and well-being.

■ REFERENCES

Ad Hoc Committee of the Harvard Medical School to Examine the Definition of Brain Death: A definition of irreversible coma. JAMA 205:337–340, 1968

Alexander S: They decide who lives, who dies. Life (9 November):102, 1962

Altman LK: Two doctors cited for work developing artificial kidney. New York Times, September 22, 2002

American Hospital Association: Management Advisory: Ethics Committees. Chicago, IL, American Hospital Association, 1990

Aulisio MP, Arnold RM, Youngner SJ: Health care ethics consultation: nature, goals, and competencies. A position paper from the Society for Health and Human Values—Society for Bioethics Consultation Task Force on Standards for Bioethics Consultation. Ann Intern Med 133:59–69, 2000

Beecher HK: Ethics and clinical research. N Engl J Med 274:1354–1360, 1966

Fletcher JC, Lombardo PA, Marshall MF, et al. (eds): Introduction to Clinical Ethics, 2nd Edition. Hagerstown, MD, University Publishing Group, 1997

Katz J: The Nuremberg Code and the Nuremberg Trial. JAMA 276:1662–1666, 1996

National Commission for the Protection of Human Subjects of Biomedical and Behavioral Research: The Belmont Report: Ethical Principles and Guidelines for the Protection of Human Subjects of Research. Washington, DC, U.S. Government Printing Office, 1979

President's Commission for the Study of Ethical Problems in Medicine and Biomedical and Biobehavioral Research: Deciding to Forgo Life-Sustaining Treatment: A Report on the Ethical, Medical and Legal Issues in Treatment Decisions. Washington, DC, U.S. Government Printing Office, 1983

Ross JW: Handbook for Hospital Ethics Committees. Chicago, IL, American Hospital Publishing, 1986

Ross JW, Glaser JM, Rasinski-Gregory D, et al: Health Care Ethics Committees: The Next Generation. Chicago, IL, American Hospital Publishing, 1993

Teel KA: The physician's dilemma; a doctor's view: what the law should be. Baylor Law Review 27:6–9, 1975

Appendix

CASES FOR DISCUSSION

■ CASE 1

Frank Florence, a 65-year-old man with a long-standing history of bipolar affective disorder (bipolar I—manic type), end-stage chronic obstructive pulmonary disease, and coronary artery disease, is admitted to the hospital for acute and chronic respiratory failure. This is his fourth admission in the past 6 months, and in the past 3 months he has not spent more than 8 days at home. He has been on home oxygen for the past 13 years and has chronic and progressively worsening hypercarbia ($pCO_2 = 90$ torr) and hypoxemia ("good" pO_2's in the 50s with 4–6 L/min nasal O_2). He has gross anasarca, massive peripheral edema, and multivalvular heart disease with cardiomyopathy and huge cardiomegaly. He has recently been reevaluated by cardiology, pulmonology, and nephrology for any ideas for removing the fluid buildup, which has been resistant to aggressive diuresis. The consensus is that Mr. Florence is receiving maximal and optimal therapies and that there is nothing else to offer. His psychiatrist concurs.

Mr. Florence and his large family have been satisfied with this pronouncement and have been appreciative of the care he has received. There has never been any discord among the patient, his family, and his doctor, and they have agreed on most of his therapies and plan of treatment and care. Mr. Florence is decisionally capable at this time, and he is not experiencing significant psychiatric symptoms. He has declared a "limited code" directive in regard to his care that includes assisted breathing with oxygen by forced ventilation with a face mask, vasopressors, and antiarrhythmics—but no defibrillation, endotracheal tube, or mechanical ventilation. He has been able to express his acceptance of his terminal condition and has spoken with his family, with the doctor in attendance, about the expectation that his death would occur soon. The family confides that they are surprised he's lived the past couple of years.

But just before the current admission, Mr. Florence had decided that he wanted to remarry his divorced wife (and the mother of their seven children) of 40 years, although she has not agreed to it. He would like to have another couple of months to try to convince her, and then his life would be complete. He has pictures of her as a young woman at his bedside. He is sleeping poorly. He has an elated mood and is uncharacteristically irritable. With this certainty of purpose, he changes his mind about code status and requests that everything possible be done, including demanding that a cardiovascular surgeon be notified of his admission so that he can be considered for a heart transplant. The consultants again become involved, and there is consensus that the patient's desire to change treatment is preposterous, that there is no chance for the patient's long-term survival even if he were to survive resuscitation efforts. Notwithstanding, Mr. Florence continues to insist that "everything" be done. His family is excited that their father has seemingly "turned an important psychological corner," and they support him in his decision. They seem agitated with what they perceive as a negative, too-cautious attitude by the entire medical team.

* * *

What are the psychiatric and medical considerations in this case? What appropriate standards of care are relevant to this patient's situation? How do you proceed? Do you feel that these demands are reasonable? Should you try to change their minds, or have someone else try? What role might a patient care ethics committee play in this circumstance? What role might a mental health professional play in assisting this patient and family?

■ CASE 2

James Coulter is an 87-year-old gentleman with dementia of the Alzheimer's type whom you have been following for several years. His only other significant health problem is chronic obstructive pulmonary disease—a result of a more than 70-pack-per-year smoking history, although he stopped smoking 10 years ago. For the past year, his dementia has progressively worsened, and he is now completely dependent on his wife of 57 years. He cannot remember his name or his wife's name and cannot repeat any of three objects immediately after you name them to him. He previously executed a living will and named his wife as attorney-in-fact in his durable power of attorney for health care; she is acting as his legal surrogate.

Last week, after his son's wife moved into the house to help with his care, Mr. Coulter fell while getting out of a chair and broke three ribs on his right side, causing a 50% pneumothorax. He was hospitalized and a chest tube was placed. He developed pneumonia while in the hospital and required aggressive management with oxygen given by face mask (though he never required ventilator support), antibiotics, frequent suctioning, and intravenous hydration. He was stuporous for several days, then awakened somewhat but would not eat or take anything by mouth. After a week in the hospital, the chest tube was removed, the pneumonia showed evidence of resolving, and he was found to be adequately hydrated, with normal lab values, including electrolytes.

At this point, a family conference was held to consider nasogastric feeding and subsequent care. A nursing home bed had become available. Mrs. Coulter reminded the family that her husband had desired never to have long-term, high-technology care and had specifically stated that he never wanted to be on a ventilator. Because of his confusion, she felt that a nasogastric, or enteral, tube for feeding and nutrition was out of the question. The entire family agreed with her judgment, calling such treatment "cruel" and "the last thing in the world he would ever want." A decision was made to discontinue intravenous fluids but to offer as much care as possible in the nursing home, with careful administration of oral fluids and medicines by mouth without restarting intravenous lines. Mr. Coulter was discharged to the nursing home after approximately 2 weeks in the hospital, 4 days after intravenous fluids were discontinued.

After only a couple of days in the nursing home, you receive a frantic call from Mrs. Coulter. She says that the doctor in the nursing home has just seen her husband and has expressed profound concerns about dehydration, mentioning that his "sodium is probably out of whack." The family has changed its cumulative decision and wants Mr. Coulter readmitted to the hospital with intravenous fluids restarted and a nasogastric tube inserted. They feel that he was discharged too soon, and they are dissatisfied with the care provided in the nursing home.

* * *

What are the medical issues at this time? What standards of care are relevant in this patient's care? What do you understand about the patient's preferences and values? How do you manage the request voiced by Mrs. Coulter? Is it right to resume care that was considered an assault just a few days ago? How would you involve the ethics committee of your hospital, or otherwise find a resource for the ethical discussions required for this situation? What role might a mental health professional play in assisting this family?

■ CASE 3

Brenda and Frank Foot have been married for the past 48 years. They have three grown children with families of their own in the area. They both retired from work several years ago because of worsening health, but have enjoyed their time together despite increasing debilities.

They both have severe chronic lung disease and continue to smoke cigarettes. About 2 years ago, Mrs. Foot had a severe myocardial infarction from which her doctors and family feared she would not recover. Serious discussions were initiated about what type of life support and resuscitation should be performed if needed. The family was deeply disturbed that her preferences were not better known. Mrs. Foot did surprisingly well, however, and after rehabilitation returned to her normal activities. However, she adamantly refused any further discussion of her illness or of advance directives.

Mr. Foot was actually much sicker than his wife. He had already had two heart attacks, had undergone several hospitalizations in the past year for congestive heart failure, and his lung disease had worsened. He now was house confined, on chronic oxygen, and was being visited by home health regularly. Mr. Foot recognized his deteriorating condition and spoke to his wife about his wishes for future health care, although she was uncomfortable with these subjects. He made out a living will, completed an advance directive that excluded ventilator use, named Mrs. Foot as attorney-in-fact in the durable power of attorney for health care, and told her that if his condition drastically worsened, he did not want to be sent to the hospital.

But his condition did drastically worsen, on the day the lawyer came and took the directives "downtown" to be notarized. Despite the recent conversations, Mrs. Foot telephoned the rescue squad and then returned to her husband's bedside. He told her that he loved her, reminded her of the living will, and then seemed to fall asleep, although he continued to show labored breathing. The rescue squad arrived, placed an endotracheal tube to assist breathing, and took Mr. Foot to the emergency department, where he was attached to a ventilator and quickly moved to the ICU.

He has now been on the ventilator in the ICU for 9 days. He has not awakened but does respond to pinches and to shouts occasionally. Mrs. Foot says his care "could not have been better—they've done everything and then some." But she eventually confides to her family and to the doctors about their conversations and the advance directives. She asks the doctors for help with the decision about what to do, but also requests that they "do everything possible to make him comfortable—I couldn't watch him suffer." She then regroups with her family, who are confused and do not understand why she wants continued support in light of the preferences Mr. Foot had expressed about his care.

*   *   *

What are the medical issues in the case? What standards of care are relevant to this patient's current situation? What should the response of the physicians be? Of the nurses in the ICU? Could an ethics committee help in your hospital with this? What role might a mental health professional play in helping to address this situation?

Appendix A

GLOSSARY

Altruism   Altruism represents the commitment to help others, setting aside self-interest and at times requiring self-sacrifice.

Autonomy   Autonomy is the capacity to make authentic, reasoned decisions for oneself.

Beneficence   Beneficence represents the commitment to act in a manner that brings about 'good outcomes' or benefit.

Compassion   Compassion is the genuine regard for the experience and suffering of another person, often including a response intended to provide kindness and comfort for that individual.

Confidentiality   Confidentiality is the obligation not to disclose information obtained from a patient, or information gathered through observation in caring for a patient, without his or her permission. In our society, confidentiality is identified as a privilege that may be overruled by important legal considerations.

Fidelity   Fidelity represents the dedicated commitment to serving the well-being and best interests of the patient.

Honesty   Honesty represents the duty to be truthful, involving the positive obligation to convey information and impressions accurately as well as the negative obligation to not mislead or deceive through omissions of the truth.

Justice   Justice represents the fair, equitable distribution of benefits and burdens in society.

Nonmaleficence   Nonmaleficence represents the obligation to avoid doing harm.

Respect for persons   Respect for persons represents fundamental regard for the worth and dignity of a human person.

Therapeutic boundaries   Therapeutic boundaries are practices that help structure professional relationships so that they foster the well-being and benefit of the patient, separating professional therapeutic relationships from other kinds of personal interactions.

Appendix B

ADDITIONAL READINGS

Chapter 1. Ethics: Principles and Professionalism

American Medical Association Council on Ethical and Judicial Affairs: Code of Medical Ethics: Current Opinions With Annotations, 2002–2003 Edition. Chicago, IL, American Medical Association, 2002

Beauchamp TL, Childress JF: Principles of Biomedical Ethics, 5th Edition. New York, Oxford University Press, 2001

Bloch S, Chodoff P, Green SA (eds): Psychiatric Ethics, 3rd Edition. Oxford, UK, Oxford University Press, 1999

Boyd KM, Higgs R, Pinching AJ: The New Dictionary of Medical Ethics. London, BMJ Publishing, 1997

Churchill LR: Beneficence, in Encyclopedia of Bioethics, Revised Edition. Edited by Reich WT. New York, Macmillan, 1995, pp 243–247

Dickenson D, Fulford B, Fulford KWM: In Two Minds: A Casebook of Psychiatric Ethics. Oxford, UK, Oxford University Press, 2000

Dyer AR: Ethics and Psychiatry: Toward Professional Definition. Washington, DC, American Psychiatric Press, 1998

Frankena WR: Ethics. Englewood Cliffs, NJ, Prentice Hall Professional Technical Reference, 1963

Guttentag OE: On defining medicine. The Christian Scholar 46:200–211, 1963

Hebert PC: Doing Right: A Practical Guide to Ethics for Medical Trainees and Physicians. Oxford, UK, Oxford University Press, 1995

Jonsen AR, Siegler M, Winslade WJ: Clinical Ethics, 4th Edition. New York, McGraw-Hill, 1998

Jonsen AR, Walters L, Veatch RM: Sourcebook in Bioethics. Washington, DC, Georgetown University Press, 2000

Kass LR: Professing ethically. On the place of ethics in defining medicine. JAMA 249:1305–1310, 1983

Koocher GP, Keith-Spiegel PC (eds): Ethics in Psychology: Professional Standards and Cases, 2nd Edition. Oxford, UK, Oxford University Press, 1998

LaCombe MA: On professionalism. Am J Med 94:329, 1993

Lo B: Resolving Ethical Dilemmas: A Guide for Clinicians, 2nd Edition. Philadelphia, PA, Lippincott Williams & Wilkins, 2000

Racy J: Professionalism: sane and insane [editorial]. J Clin Psychiatry 51: 138–140, 1990

Reynolds PP: Reaffirming professionalism through the education community [see comments]. Ann Intern Med 120:609–614, 1994

Simon RI: Clinical Psychiatry and the Law, 2nd Edition. Washington, DC, American Psychiatric Press, 1992

Sterba JP: Justice, in Encyclopedia of Bioethics, Revised Edition. Edited by Reich WT. New York, Macmillan, 1995, pp 1308–1315

Stobo JD, Blank LL: American Board of Internal Medicine's Project Professionalism: staying ahead of the wave. Am J Med 97:1–3, 1994

Toulmin SE, Jonsen AR: The Abuse of Casuistry: A History of Moral Reasoning. Berkeley, CA, University of California Press, 1990

Chapter 2. Clinical Decision-Making and Ethics Skills

Bernstein BE, Hartsell T: The Portable Ethicist for Mental Health Professionals. New York, Wiley, 2000

Bradley E, Walker L, Blechner B, et al: Assessing capacity to participate in discussions of advance directives in nursing homes: findings from a study of the Patient Self Determination Act. J Am Geriatr Soc 45:79–83, 1997

Grimes AL, McCullough LB, Kunik ME, et al: Informed consent and neuroanatomic correlates of intentionality and voluntariness among psychiatric patients. Psychiatr Serv 51:1561–1567, 2000

Guttentag OE: On defining medicine. The Christian Scholar 46:200–211, 1963

Humber JM, Almeder RF: Alternative Medicine and Ethics. Biomedical Ethics Reviews. Totowa, NJ, Humana Press, 1998

Hundert EM: A model for ethical problem solving in medicine, with practical applications. Am J Psychiatry 144:839–846, 1987

Jonsen AR, Siegler M, Winslade WJ: Clinical Ethics, 4th Edition. New York, McGraw-Hill, 1998

Kushner TK, Thomasma DC: Ward Ethics: Dilemmas for Medical Students and Doctors in Training. Oxford, UK, Cambridge University Press, 2001

Lakin M: Coping With Ethical Dilemmas in Psychotherapy. New York, Pergamon, 1991

Morenz B, Sales B: Complexity of ethical decision making in psychiatry. Ethics Behav 7(1):1–14, 1997

Moser DJ, Schultz SK, Arndt S, et al: Capacity to provide informed consent for participation in schizophrenia and HIV research. Am J Psychiatry 159:1201–1207, 2002

Okasha A, Arboleda-Florez J, Sartorius N: Ethics, Culture, and Psychiatry: International Perspectives. Washington, DC, American Psychiatric Press, 2000

O'Rourke K: A Primer for Health Care Ethics: Essays for a Pluralistic Society, 2nd Edition. Washington, DC, Georgetown University Press, 2000

Roberts LW: Informed consent and the capacity for voluntarism. Am J Psychiatry 159:705–712, 2002

Roberts LW, McCarty T, Roberts BB, et al: Clinical ethics teaching in psychiatric supervision. Acad Psychiatry 20:172–184, 1996

Roberts LW, Geppert CM, Bailey R: Ethics in psychiatric practice: essential ethical skills, informed consent, the therapeutic relationship, and confidentiality. Journal of Psychiatric Practice 8(5):290–305, 2002

Sadler JZ, Hulgus YF: Clinical problem solving and the biopsychosocial model. Am J Psychiatry 149:1315–1323, 1992

Weston A: A Practical Companion to Ethics. Oxford, UK, Oxford University Press, 1997

Chapter 3.   The Psychotherapeutic Relationship

American Psychiatric Association: The Principles of Medical Ethics With Annotations Applicable to Psychiatry. Washington, DC, American Psychiatric Association, 2001

Clouser KD: What is medical ethics? Ann Intern Med 80:657–660, 1974

Dyer AR, Roberts LW: Divided loyalties in health care, in Encyclopedia of Bioethics, 3rd Edition. New York, Macmillan, 2003, pp 673–677

Epstein RS, Simon RI: The Exploitation Index: an early warning indicator of boundary violations in psychotherapy. Bull Menninger Clin 54:450–465, 1990

Epstein RS, Simon RI, Kay GG: Assessing boundary violations in psychotherapy: survey results with the Exploitation Index. Bull Menninger Clin 56:150–166, 1992

Gabbard GO: Psychodynamic Psychiatry in Clinical Practice, 3rd Edition. Washington, DC, American Psychiatric Press, 2000

Knight JA: Divided loyalties in mental health care, in Encyclopedia of Bioethics, 2nd Edition. New York, Macmillan, 1995, pp 629–633

Knight JA: Divided loyalties in health care (revised by Dyer AR, Roberts LW), in Encyclopedia of Bioethics, 3rd Edition. Post SG, Editor-in-Chief. New York, Macmillan, 2003 (forthcoming)

Lakin M: Coping With Ethical Dilemmas in Psychotherapy. New York, Pergamon, 1991

Lifton RJ: Advocacy and corruption in the healing professions. International Review of Psychoanalysis 3(4):385–398, 1976

Lifton RJ: The Nazi Doctors: Medical Killing and the Psychology of Genocide. New York, Basic Books, 1986

Macklin R: Man, Mind, and Morality: The Ethics of Behavior Control. Englewood Cliffs, NJ, Prentice Hall, 1982

Malley PB, Reilly EP: Legal and Ethical Dimensions for Mental Health Professionals. Philadelphia, PA, Taylor & Francis, 1999

Murdoch I: Metaphysics as a Guide to Morals: Philosophical Reflections. New York, Viking Penguin, 1992

Roukema RW: What Every Patient, Family, Friend, and Caregiver Needs to Know About Psychiatry. Washington, DC, American Psychiatric Press, 1998

Chapter 4. Informed Consent and Decisional Capacity

Appelbaum PS, Grisso T: Assessing patients' capacities to consent to treatment. N Engl J Med 319:1635–1638, 1988

Appelbaum PS, Grisso T: The MacArthur Competence Study I, II, III. Law and Human Behavior 19:105–174, 1995

Carpenter WT Jr, Gold JM, Lahti HC, et al: Decisional capacity for informed consent in schizophrenia research [see comments]. Arch Gen Psychiatry 57:533–538, 2000

Drane JF: Competency to give an informed consent. A model for making clinical assessments. JAMA 252:925–927, 1984

Dunn LB, Jeste DV: Enhancing informed consent for research and treatment. Neuropsychopharmacology 24:595–607, 2001

Grisso T, Appelbaum PS, Hill-Fotouhi C: The MacCAT-T: A clinical tool to assess patients' capacities to make treatment decisions. Psychiatr Serv 48:1415–1419, 1999

High DM: Who will make health care decisions for me when I can't? J Aging Health 2(3):291–309, 1990

Lidz CW, Meisel A, Osterweis M, et al: Barriers to informed consent. Ann Intern Med 99:539–543, 1983

Marson DC, Ingram KK, Cody HA, et al: Assessing the competency of patients with Alzheimer's disease under different legal standards. A prototype instrument [see comments]. Arch Neurol 52:949–954, 1995

Mouton C, Teno JM, Mor V, et al: Communication of preferences for care among human immunodeficiency virus-infected patients. Barriers to informed decisions? Arch Fam Med 6:342–347, 1997

Roberts LW: Informed consent and the capacity for voluntarism. Am J Psychiatry 159:705–712, 2002

Sachs GA, Stocking CB, Stern R, et al: Ethical aspects of dementia research: informed consent and proxy consent. Clin Res 42:403–412, 1994

Stanley B, Stanley M: Psychiatric patients' comprehension of consent information. Psychopharmacol Bull 23:375–378, 1987

Sugarman J, McCrory DC, Hubal RC: Getting meaningful informed consent from older adults: a structured literature review of empirical research. J Am Geriatr Soc 46:517–524, 1998

Sugarman J, McCrory DC, Powell D, et al: Empirical research on informed consent. An annotated bibliography [see comments]. Hastings Cent Rep 29(1):S1–S42, 1999

Tomamichel M, Sessa C, Herzig S, et al: Informed consent for phase I studies: evaluation of quantity and quality of information provided to patients. Ann Oncol 6(4):363–369, 1995

Warren JW, Sobal J, Tenney JH, et al: Informed consent by proxy. An issue in research with elderly patients. N Engl J Med 315:1124–1128, 1986

Wirshing DA, Wirshing WC, Marder SR, et al: Informed consent: assessment of comprehension. Am J Psychiatry 155:1508–1511, 1998

Chapter 5.   Ethical Use of Power in High-Risk Situations

American Psychiatric Association Commission on AIDS: Position statement on confidentiality, disclosure, and protection of others. Am J Psychiatry 150:852, 1993

Anfang SA, Appelbaum PS: Twenty years after *Tarasoff*: reviewing the duty to protect. Harv Rev Psychiatry 4:67–76, 1996

Appelbaum PS, Gutheil TG: Drug refusal: a study of psychiatric inpatients. Am J Psychiatry 137:340–346, 1980

Backlar P, Cutler DE (eds): Ethics in Community Mental Health Care: Commonplace Concerns. New York, Kluwer Academic, 2002

Fawcett J: Treating impulsivity and anxiety in the suicidal patient. Ann N Y Acad Sci 932:94–102, discussion 102–105, 2001

Gardner W, Hoge SK, Bennett N, et al: Two scales for measuring patients' perceptions for coercion during mental hospital admission. Behav Sci Law 11(3):307–321, 1993

Gardner W, Lidz CW, Hoge SK, et al: Patients' revisions of their beliefs about the need for hospitalization. Am J Psychiatry 156:1385–1391, 1999

Hall RC, Platt DE: Suicide risk assessment: a review of risk factors for suicide in 100 patients who made severe suicide attempts. Evaluation of suicide risk in a time of managed care. Psychosomatics 40:18–27, 1999

Harris GT, Rice ME: Risk appraisal and management of violent behavior. Psychiatr Serv 48:1168–1176, 1997

Hickson GB, Federspiel CF, Pichert JW, et al: Patient complaints and malpractice risk. JAMA 287:2951–2957, 2002

Hiday VA, Swartz MS, Swanson JW, et al: Criminal victimization of persons with severe mental illness. Psychiatr Serv 50:62–68, 1999

Hiday VA, Swartz MS, Swanson JW, et al: Coercion in mental health care, in Ethics in Community Mental Health: Commonplace Concerns. Edited by Backlar P, Cutler DE. New York, Kluwer Academic, 2002a, pp 117–136

Hiday VA, Swartz MS, Swanson JW, et al: Impact of outpatient commitment on victimization of people with severe mental illness. Am J Psychiatry 159:1403–1411, 2002b

Hoge SK, Appelbaum PS, Lawlor T, et al: A prospective, multicenter study of patients' refusal of antipsychotic medication. Arch Gen Psychiatry 47:949–956, 1990

Link BG, Phelan JC, Bresnahan M, et al: Public conceptions of mental illness: labels, causes, dangerousness, and social distance. Am J Public Health 89:1328–1333, 1999

Malley PB, Reilly EP: Legal and Ethical Dimensions for Mental Health Professionals. Philadelphia, PA, Taylor & Francis, 1999

Maltsberger JT: Calculated risks in the treatment of intractably suicidal patients. Psychiatry 57:199–212, 1994

Marder SR, Mebane A, Chien CP, et al: A comparison of patients who refuse and consent to neuroleptic treatment. Am J Psychiatry 140:470–472, 1983

National Alliance for the Mentally Ill: NAMI statement on involuntary outpatient commitment. Am Psychol 42:571–584, 1987

National Institute of Mental Health: In Harm's Way: Suicide in America (NIH Publ No. 03-4594). Bethesda, MD, National Institute of Mental Health, 2001

Pope KS, Vasquez MJ: Ethics in Psychotherapy and Counseling. San Francisco, CA, Jossey-Bass, 1998

Roth LH, Appelbaum PS, Sallee R, et al: The dilemma of denial in the assessment of competency to refuse treatment. Am J Psychiatry 139:910–913, 1982

Schwartz III, Vingiano W, Perez CB: Autonomy and the right to refuse treatment: patients' attitudes after involuntary medication. Hosp Community Psychiatry 39:1049–1054, 1988

Simon RI: Clinical Psychiatry and the Law, 2nd Edition. Washington, DC, American Psychiatric Press, 1992

Swanson J, Estroff S, Swartz M, et al: Violence and severe mental disorder in clinical and community populations: the effects of psychotic symptoms, comorbidity, and lack of treatment. Psychiatry 60:1–22, 1997

Swanson JW, Holzer CE 3rd, Ganju VK, et al: Violence and psychiatric disorder in the community: evidence from the Epidemiologic Catchment Area surveys. Hosp Community Psychiatry 41:761–770, 1990

Swartz MS, Swanson JW, Wagner HR, et al: Can involuntary outpatient commitment reduce hospital recidivism? Findings from a randomized trial with severely mentally ill individuals. Am J Psychiatry 156:1968–1975, 1999

Szasz TS: Involuntary psychiatry. University of Cincinnati Law Review 45(3):347–365, 1976

Treatment Advocacy Center: Episodes Database. Available at: http://www.psychlaws.org/ep.asp. Accessed August 31, 2002

Chapter 6.   Confidentiality and Truth Telling

Allen LB, Glicken AD, Beach RK, et al: Adolescent health care experience of gay, lesbian, and bisexual young adults. J Adolesc Health 23:212–220, 1998

American Medical Association Council on Ethical and Judicial Affairs: Code of Medical Ethics: Current Opinions With Annotations, 2002–2003 Edition. Chicago, IL, American Medical Association, 2002

Baylis P: Medical negligence. Trans Med Soc Lond 89:75–80, 1973

Blackhall LJ, Frank G, Murphy S, et al: Bioethics in a different tongue: the case of truth-telling. J Urban Health 78:59–71, 2001

Cheng TL, Savageau JA, Sattler AL, et al: Confidentiality in health care. A survey of knowledge, perceptions, and attitudes among high school students [see comments]. JAMA 269:1404–1407, 1993

Cogswell BE: Cultivating the trust of adolescent patients. Fam Med 17:254–258, 1985

Fletcher JC: Commentary: Ethics is everybody's business, especially in regard to confidentiality. Journal of Clinical Ethics 2(1):30–31, 1991

Gert B, Culver CM, Clouser KD: Confidentiality, in Bioethics: A Return to Fundamentals. New York, Oxford University Press, 1997, pp 181–194

Hippocratic Writings. Translated by Chadwick J, Mann WN. New York, Penguin Books, 1950

Lindenthal JJ, Thomas CS: Psychiatrists, the public, and confidentiality. J Nerv Ment Dis 170:319–323, 1982

Miyaji N: The power of compassion: truth-telling among American doctors in the care of dying patients. Soc Sci Med 36:249–264, 1993

Novack DH, Detering BJ, Arnold R, et al: Physicians' attitudes toward using deception to resolve difficult ethical problems. JAMA 261:2980–2985, 1989

Pope KS, Vetter VA: Ethical dilemmas encountered by members of the American Psychological Association: a national survey. Am Psychol 47:397–411, 1992

Price AR: Anonymity and pseudonymity in whistleblowing to the U.S. Office of Research Integrity. Acad Med 73:467–472, 1998

Roback HB, Moore RF, Bloch FS, et al: Confidentiality in group psychotherapy: empirical findings and the law. Int J Group Psychother 46:117–135, 1996

Roberts LW, Battaglia J, Smithpeter M, et al: An office on main street: health care dilemmas in small communities. Hastings Cent Rep 29(4):28–37, 1999

Roberts LW, Geppert C, Bailey R: Ethics in psychiatric practice: essential ethics skills, informed consent, the therapeutic relationship, and confidentiality. Journal of Psychiatric Practice 8(5):290–305, 2002

Rubin SB, Zoloth L: Margin of Error: The Ethics of Mistakes in the Practice of Medicine. Hagerstown, MD, University Publishing Group, 2000

Siegler M: Sounding boards. Confidentiality in medicine—a decrepit concept. N Engl J Med 307:1518–1521, 1982

Sweet MP, Bernat JL: A study of the ethical duty of physicians to disclose errors. J Clin Ethics 8:341–348, 1997

Ubel PA, Zell MM, Miller DJ, et al: Elevator talk: observational study of inappropriate comments in a public space. Am J Med 99:190–194, 1995

Ullom-Minnich PD, Kallail KJ: Physicians' strategies for safeguarding confidentiality: the influence of community and practice characteristics. J Fam Pract 37:445–448, 1993

Weiss BD: Confidentiality expectations of patients, physicians, and medical students. JAMA 247:2695–2697, 1982

Wettstein RM: Confidentiality, in American Psychiatric Press Review of Psychiatry, Vol 13. Edited by Oldham JM, Riba MB. Washington, DC, American Psychiatric Press, 1994, pp 343–364

Chapter 7. Caring for Children

Statutory Chapters in New Mexico Statutes Annotated (NMSA) 1978; Chapter 32A Children's Code, Article 6 Children's Mental Health and Developmental Disabilities, 32A-6-14 Treatment and Habilitation of Children; Liability (1995).

Annie E. Casey Foundation: Kids Count data book. Baltimore, MD, Annie E. Casey Foundation, 2000

Blustein J, Levine C, Dubler NN: The Adolescent Alone: Decisionmaking in Health Care in the United States. Cambridge, UK, Cambridge University Press, 1999

Boonstra H, Nash E: Minors and the right to consent to health care. The Guttmacher Report on Public Policy 3(4):4–8, 2000

DeKraai MB, Sales BD: Liability in child therapy and research. J Consult Clin Psychol 59:853–860, 1991

Green AH: Victims of child abuse, in American Psychiatric Press Review of Psychiatry, Vol 13. Edited by Oldham JM, Riba MB. Washington, DC, American Psychiatric Press, 1994, pp 589–609

Hoagwood K, Jensen PS, Fisher CB (eds): Ethical Issues in Mental Health Research With Children and Adolescents. Mahwah, NJ, Lawrence Erlbaum, 1996

Jellinek MS, Little M, Benedict K, et al: Placement outcomes of 206 severely maltreated children in the Boston Juvenile Court system: a 7.5-year follow-up study. Child Abuse Negl 19:1051–1064, 1995

Jonsen AR, Siegler M, Winslade WJ: Clinical Ethics, 4th Edition. New York, McGraw-Hill, 1998

Koocher GP, Keith-Spiegel PC: Children, Ethics and the Law. Lincoln, NE, University of Nebraska Press, 1990

Malley PB, Reilly EP: Legal and Ethical Dimensions for Mental Health Professionals. Philadelphia, PA, Taylor & Francis, 1999

Mannheim CI, Sancilio M, Phipps-Yonas S, et al: Ethical ambiguities in the practice of child clinical psychology. Professional Psychology: Research and Practice 33:24–29, 2002

Martin A, Kaufman J, Charney D: Pharmacotherapy of early onset depression. Update and new directions. Child Adolesc Psychiatr Clin North Am 9:135–157, 2000

Melton GB: Parents and children: legal reform to facilitate children's participation. Am Psychol 54:935–944, 1999

Munir K, Earls F: Ethical principles governing research in child and adolescent psychiatry [see comments]. J Am Acad Child Adolesc Psychiatry 31:408–414, 1992

National Institutes of Health: NIH Policy and Guidelines on the Inclusion of Children as Participants in Research Involving Human Subjects. Bethesda, MD, National Institutes of Health, 1998

Ondrusek N, Abramovitch R, Pencharz P, et al: Empirical examination of the ability of children to consent to clinical research. J Med Ethics 24:158–165, 1998

Rosato J: The ethics of clinical trials: a child's view. J Law Med Ethics 28:362–378, 2000

Sedlak AJ, Broadhurst DD: Third National Incidence Study of Child Abuse and Neglect. Washington, DC, U.S. Department of Health and Human Services, Administration for Children and Families, Administration on Children, Youth and Families, National Center on Child Abuse and Neglect, 1996

U.S. Department of Health and Human Services: Code of Federal Regulations, Title 45: Public Welfare. Part 46: Protection of Human Subjects Regulation Governing Protections Afforded Children in Research (Subpart D). Washington, DC, U.S. Department of Health and Human Services, 1983

U.S. Department of Health and Human Services: Report of the Surgeon General's Conference on Children's Mental Health: A National Action Agenda. Washington, DC, U.S. Department of Health and Human Services, 2000

Vitiello B: Ethical considerations in psychopharmacological research involving children and adolescents. J Clin Psychopharmacol 171:86–91, 2003

Chapter 8.   Caring for People With Addictions

Abide MM, Richards HC, Ramsay SG: Moral reasoning and consistency of belief and behavior: decisions about substance abuse. J Drug Educ 31:367–384, 2001

Brody JL, Waldron HB: Ethical issues on the treatment of adolescent substance abuse disorders. Addict Behav 25:217–228, 2000

Buchanan D, Khoshnood K, Stopka T, et al: Ethical dilemmas created by the criminalization of status behaviors: case examples from ethnographic field research with injection drug users. Health Educ Behav 29:30–42, 2002

Gerstein DR, Johnson RA, Larison CL: Alcohol and Drug Treatment Outcomes for Patients and Welfare Recipients: Outcomes, Benefits, and Costs. Washington, DC, U.S. Department of Health and Human Services, Office of the Secretary for Planning and Evaluation, 1997

Harris EC, Barraclough B: Excess mortality of mental disorder. Br J Psychiatry 173:11–53, 1998

Kessler RC, McGonagle KA, Zhao S, et al: Lifetime and 12-month prevalence of DSM-III-R psychiatric disorders in the United States. Results from the National Comorbidity Survey. Arch Gen Psychiatry 51:8–19, 1994

Link BG, Struening EL, Rahav M, et al: On stigma and its consequences: evidence from a longitudinal study of men with dual diagnoses of mental illness and substance abuse. J Health Soc Behav 38:177–190, 1997

Link BG, Phelan JC, Bresnahan M, et al: Public conceptions of mental illness: labels, causes, dangerousness, and social distance. Am J Public Health 89:1328–1333, 1999

Marlowe DB, Kirby KC, Bonieskie M, et al: Assessment of coercive and noncoercive pressures to enter drug abuse treatment. Drug Alcohol Depend 42:77–84, 1996

McCrady BS, Bux DA Jr: Ethical issues in informed consent with substance abusers. J Consult Clin Psychol 67:186–193, 1999

McGinnis JM, Foege WH: Mortality and morbidity attributable to use of addictive substances in the United States. Proc Assoc Am Physicians 111:109–118, 1999

McLellan AT, Lewis DC, O'Brien CP, et al: Drug dependence, a chronic medical illness: implications for treatment, insurance, and outcomes evaluation. JAMA 284:1689–1695, 2000

National Household Survey on Drug Abuse. Washington, DC, Substance Abuse and Mental Health Services Administration, 1999

Posternak MA, Mueller TI: Assessing the risks and benefits of benzodiazepines for anxiety disorders in patients with a history of substance abuse or dependence. Am J Addict 10:48–68, 2001

Regier DA, Narrow WE, Rae DS, et al: The de facto US mental and addictive disorders service system. Epidemiologic Catchment Area prospective 1-year prevalence rates of disorders and services. Arch Gen Psychiatry 50:85–94, 1993

Rice DP, Kelman S, Miller LS: Estimates of economic costs of alcohol and drug abuse and mental illness, 1985 and 1988. Public Health Rep 106:280–292, 1991

Single E, Rehm J, Robson L, et al: The relative risks and etiologic fractions of different causes of death and disease attributable to alcohol, tobacco and illicit drug use in Canada. CMAJ 162:1669–1675, 2000

Chapter 9.   Caring for "Difficult" People

Drossman DA: The problem patient: evaluation and care of medical patients with psychosocial disturbances. Ann Intern Med 88:366–372, 1978

Gross R, Olfson M, Gameroff M, et al: Borderline personality disorder in primary care. Arch Intern Med 162:53–60, 2002

Hahn SR, Kroenke K, Spitzer RL, et al: The difficult patient: prevalence, psychopathology, and functional impairment. J Gen Intern Med 11:1–8, 1996

Hahn SR, Thompson KS, Wills TA, et al: The difficult doctor-patient relationship: somatization, personality and psychopathology. J Clin Epidemiol 47:647–657, 1994

Jackson JL, Kroenke K: Difficult patient encounters in the ambulatory clinic: clinical predictors and outcomes. Arch Intern Med 159:1069–1075, 1999

McCarty T, Roberts LW: The difficult patient, in Medicine: A Primary Care Approach. Edited by Rubin RH, Voss C, Derksen DJ, et al. Philadelphia, PA, WB Saunders, 1996, pp 395–399

Robbins JM, Beck PR, Mueller DP, et al: Therapists' perceptions of difficult psychiatric patients. J Nerv Ment Dis 176:490–497, 1988

Schafer S, Nowlis DP: Personality disorders among difficult patients. Arch Fam Med 7:126–129, 1998

Sharpe M, Mayou R, Seagroatt V, et al: Why do doctors find some patients difficult to help? Q J Med 87:187–193, 1994

Valliant GE: The beginning of wisdom is never calling a patient a borderline; or, the clinical management of immature defenses in the treatment of individuals with personality disorders. J Psychother Pract Res 1:117–134, 1992

Woolley D, Clements T: Family medicine residents' and community physicians' concerns about patient truthfulness. Acad Med 72:155–157, 1997

Wright AL, Morgan WJ: On the creation of "problem" patients. Soc Sci Med 30:951–959, 1990

Chapter 10. Caring for People in Small Communities

Braden J, Beauregard K: Health status and access to care of rural and urban populations. National Medical Expenditure Survey Research Findings 18 (AHCPR Publ No. 94-0031). Rockville, MD, Agency for Health Care Policy and Research, 1994

Henderson G, King NMP, Strauss RP, et al. (eds): The Social Medicine Reader. Durham, NC, Duke University Press, 1997

Niemira DA: Grassroots grappling: ethics committees at rural hospitals. Ann Intern Med 109:981–983, 1988

Perkins DV, Hudson BL, Gray DM, et al: Decisions and justifications by community mental health providers about hypothetical ethical dilemmas. Psychiatr Serv 49:1317–1322, 1998

Roberts LW, Battaglia J, Epstein RS: Frontier ethics: mental health care needs and ethical dilemmas. Psychiatr Serv 50:497–503, 1999

Roberts LW, Battaglia J, Smithpeter M, et al: An office on main street: health care dilemmas in small communities. Hastings Cent Rep 29:28–37, 1999

Roberts LW, Monaghan-Geernaert P, Battaglia J, Warner TD: Personal health care attitudes of rural clinicians: a preliminary study of 127 multidisciplinary health care providers in Alaska and New Mexico. Rural Mental Health 28(1), 2003

Simon RI: Treatment boundary violations: clinical, ethical, and legal considerations. Bull Am Acad Psychiatry Law 20:269–288, 1992

Simon RI, Williams IC: Maintaining treatment boundaries in small communities and rural areas. Psychiatr Serv 50:1440–1446, 1999

Turner LN, Marquis K, Burman ME: Rural nurse practitioners: perceptions of ethical dilemmas. J Am Acad Nurse Pract 8:269–274, 1996

Ullom-Minnich PD, Kallail KJ: Physicians' strategies for safeguarding confidentiality: the influence of community and practice characteristics. J Fam Pract 37:445–448, 1993

Wagenfeld MO, Murray JD, Mohatt DF, et al: Mental Health and Rural America: 1980–1993. An Overview and Annotated Bibliography. Washington, DC, Office of Rural Health Policy, Health Resources and Services Administration, National Institutes of Health, and Public Health Service, 1994

Chapter 11. Caring for People at End of Life

Academy of Psychosomatic Medicine: Position Statement: Psychiatric Aspects of Excellent End of Life Care, 1998–1999. Available at: www.apm.org\eol-care.html. Accessed August 31, 2002

Becker E: The Denial of Death. New York, Free Press, 1973

Breitbart W, Lintz K: Psychiatric issues in the care of dying patients, in Textbook of Consultation-Liaison Psychiatry: Psychiatry in the Medically Ill, 2nd Edition. Edited by Wise MG, Rundell JR. Washington, DC, American Psychiatric Press, 2002, pp 771–806

Burt RA: The medical futility debate: patient choice, physician obligation, and end-of-life care. J Palliat Med 5:249–254, 2002

Byrock I: Dying Well: Peace and Possibilities at the End of Life. New York, Riverhead Books, 1997

Ganzini L, Lee MA, Heintz RT, et al: The effect of depression treatment on elderly patients' preferences for life-sustaining medical therapy. Am J Psychiatry 151:1631–1636, 1994

Gibson JM, Lambert P, Nathanson P: The values history: an innovation in surrogate medical decision-making. Law, Medicine, and Health Care 18(3):202–212, 1990

Kubler-Ross E: Death and Dying. New York, Macmillan, 1970

Lo B, Quill T, Tulsky J: Discussing palliative care with patients. Ann Intern Med 130:744–749, 1999

Quill TE: Initiating end-of-life discussions with seriously ill patients: addressing the "elephant in the room." JAMA 284:2502–2507, 2000

Puchalski CM: Spirituality and end-of-life care: a time for listening and caring. J Palliat Med 5:289–294, 2002

Puchalski CM, Romer AL: Taking a spiritual history allows clinicians to understand patients more fully. J Palliat Med 3:129–137, 2000

Roberts LW, Muskin PR, Warner TD, et al: Attitudes of consultation liaison psychiatrists toward physician assisted death practices. Psychosomatics 38:459–471, 1997

Roberts LW, Roberts BB, Warner TD, et al: Internal medicine, psychiatry, and emergency medicine residents' views of assisted death practices. Arch Intern Med 157:1603–1609, 1997

Steinberg MD, Youngner SJ (eds): End-of-Life Decisions: A Psychosocial Perspective. Washington, DC, American Psychiatric Press, 1998

Steinhauser KE, Chistrakis NA, Cliff EC, et al: Factors considered important at the end of life by patients, family, physicians, and other care providers. JAMA 284:2476–2482, 2000

Chapter 12.   Ethical Issues in Psychiatric Genetics

Armstrong K, Calzone K, Stopfer J, et al: Factors associated with decisions about clinical BRCA1/2 testing. Cancer Epidemiol Biomarkers Prev 9:1251–1254, 2000

Billings PR, Kohn MA, de Cuevas M, et al: Discrimination as a consequence of genetic testing. Am J Hum Genet 50:476–482, 1992

Bonvicini KA: The art of recruitment: the foundation of family and linkage studies of psychiatric illness. Fam Process 37:153–165, 1998

Deftos LJ: The evolving duty to disclose the presence of genetic disease to relatives. Acad Med 73:962–968, 1998

Faraone S, Tsuang M, Tsuang D: Genetics of Mental Disorders: A Guide for Students, Clinicians, and Researchers. New York, Guilford, 1999

Holtzman NA: Primary care physicians as providers of frontline genetic services. Fetal Diagn Ther 8 (suppl 1):213–219, 1993

Jamison KR: Manic-depressive illness, genes, and creativity, in Genetics and Mental Illness: Evolving Issues for Research and Society. Edited by Hall LL. New York, Plenum, 1996, pp 111–132

Lapham EV, Kozma C, Weiss JO: Genetic discrimination: perspectives of consumers. Science 274:621–624, 1996

National Institute of Mental Health Genetics Workgroup: Genetics and Mental Disorders. Bethesda, MD, National Institute of Mental Health, 1997

Schulz PM, Schulz SC, Dibble E, et al: Patient and family attitudes about schizophrenia: implications for genetic counseling. Schizophr Bull 8: 504–513, 1982

Shore D, Berg K, Wynne D, et al: Legal and ethical issues in psychiatric genetic research. Am J Med Genet 48:17–21, 1993

Smith LB, Sapers B, Reus VI, et al: Attitudes towards bipolar disorder and predictive genetic testing among patients and providers. J Med Genet 33:544–549, 1996

Stancer HC, Wagener DK: Genetic counseling: its need in psychiatry and the directions it gives for future research. Can J Psychiatry 29:289–294, 1984

Suzuki D, Knudtson P: Genethics: The Clash Between the New Genetics and Human Values. Cambridge, MA, Harvard University Press, 1990

Targum SD, Dibble ED, Davenport YB, et al: The Family Attitudes Questionnaire. Patients' and spouses' views of bipolar illness. Arch Gen Psychiatry 38:562–568, 1981

Trippitelli CL, Jamison KR, Folstein MF, et al: Pilot study on patients' and spouses' attitudes toward potential genetic testing for bipolar disorder. Am J Psychiatry 155:899–904, 1998

Wertz DC, Fletcher JC: Ethical problems in prenatal diagnosis: a cross-cultural survey of medical geneticists in 18 nations. Prenat Diagn 9(3):145–157, 1989

Wong JG, Lieh-Mak F: Genetic discrimination and mental illness: a case report. J Med Ethics 27:393–397, 2001

Chapter 13. Ethical Issues in Managed and Evolving Systems of Care

Andreasen NC, Black DW: Introductory Textbook of Psychiatry. Washington, DC, American Psychiatric Press, 2001

Billi JE, Wise CG, Bills EA, et al: Potential effects of managed care on specialty practice at a university medical center [see comments]. N Engl J Med 333:979–983, 1995

Green SA: Is managed care ethical? Gen Hosp Psychiatry 21:256–259, 1999

Hall RC: Ethical and legal implications of managed care. Gen Hosp Psychiatry 19:200–208, 1997

Johnson JG, Spitzer RL, Williams JB, et al: Psychiatric comorbidity, health status, and functional impairment associated with alcohol abuse and dependence in primary care patients: findings of the PRIME MD-1000 study. J Consult Clin Psychol 63:133–140, 1995

Kamerow DB: Research on mental disorders in primary care settings: rationale, topics, and support. Fam Pract Res J 6:5–11, 1986

Kessler RC, McGonagle KA, Zhao S, et al: Lifetime and 12-month prevalence of DSM-III-R psychiatric disorders in the United States. Results from the National Comorbidity Survey. Arch Gen Psychiatry 51:8–19, 1994

Kralewski JE, Hart G, Perlmutter C, et al: Can academic medical centers compete in a managed care system? Acad Med 70:867–872, 1995

McCurdy L, Goode LD, Inui TS, et al: Fulfilling the social contract between medical schools and the public. Acad Med 72:1063–1070, 1997

Mechanic RE, Dobson A: The impact of managed care on clinical research: a preliminary investigation. Health Aff (Millwood) 15:72–89, 1996

Medical professionalism in the new millennium: a physician charter. ABIM Foundation (American Board of Internal Medicine); ACP-ASIM Foundation (American College of Physicians–American Society of Internal Medicine); European Federation of Internal Medicine. Ann Intern Med 136:243–246, 2002

Meyer M, Genel M, Altman RD, et al: Clinical research: assessing the future in a changing environment; summary report of conference sponsored by the American Medical Association Council on Scientific Affairs, Washington, DC, March 1996. Am J Med 104:264–271, 1998

Murray JL, Lopez AD (eds): The Global Burden of Disease. A Comprehensive Assessment of Mortality and Disability From Diseases, Injuries, and Risk Factors in 1990 and Projected to 2020. Cambridge, MA, Harvard School of Public Health, 1996

Olfson M, Fireman B, Weissman MM, et al: Mental disorders and disability among patients in a primary care group practice. Am J Psychiatry 154: 1734–1740, 1997

Penn DL, Martin J: The stigma of severe mental illness: some potential solutions for a recalcitrant problem. Psychiatr Q 69:235–247, 1998

Regier DA, Narrow WE, Rae DS, et al: The de facto US mental and addictive disorders service system. Epidemiologic Catchment Area prospective 1-year prevalence rates of disorders and services. Arch Gen Psychiatry 50:85–94, 1993

Riba M, Tasman A: Investor-owned psychiatric hospitals and universities: can their marriage succeed? Hosp Community Psychiatry 44:547–550, 1993

Roberts LW, Fraser K, Quinn D, et al: Persons with mental illness, in Managed Care: Financial, Legal, and Ethical Issues. Edited by Bennahum DA. Cleveland, OH, Pilgrim Press, 1999, pp 184–208

Sabin J: Is managed care ethical? in Controversies in Managed Mental Health Care. Edited by Lazarus A. Washington, DC, American Psychiatric Press, 1996, pp 115–128

Spitzer RL, Kroenke K, Linzer M, et al: Health-related quality of life in primary care patients with mental disorders. Results from the PRIME-MD 1000 Study. JAMA 274:1511–1517, 1995

Tanielian TL, Pincus HA, Olfson M, et al: General hospital discharges of patients with mental and physical disorders. Psychiatr Serv 48:311, 1997

U.S. Department of Health and Human Services: Mental Health: A Report of the Surgeon General. Rockville, MD, U.S. Department of Health and Human Services, 1999

Chapter 14. Ethical Issues in Clinician Health

Ingelfinger FJ: Arrogance. N Engl J Med 303:1507–1511, 1980

Miller NM, McGowen RK: The painful truth: physicians are not invincible. South Med J 93:966–973, 2000

Roberts LW, Warner TD, Carter D, et al: Caring for medical students as patients: access to services and care-seeking practices of 1,027 students at nine medical schools. Collaborative Research Group on Medical Student Healthcare. Acad Med 75:272–277, 2000

Roberts LW, Warner TD, Lyketsos C, et al: Perceptions of academic vulnerability associated with personal illness: a study of 1,027 students at nine medical schools. Collaborative Research Group on Medical Student Health. Compr Psychiatry 42:1–15, 2001

Sotile MO, Sotile WM: The Medical Marriage: A Couple's Survival Guide. New York, Carol Publishing, 1996

Stoudemire A, Rhoads JM: When the doctor needs a doctor: special considerations for the physician-patient. Ann Intern Med 98(5 pt 1):654–659, 1983

Chapter 15. Ethical Issues in Clinical Training

Accreditation Council for Graduate Medical Education: ACGME duty hours standards now in effect for all residency programs. July 1, 2003. Available at: http://www.acgme.org. Accessed December 12, 2003

American Medical Association Council on Ethical and Judicial Affairs: Code of Medical Ethics: Current Opinions With Annotations, 2002–2003 Edition. Chicago, IL, American Medical Association, 2002

Baldwin DC Jr, Daugherty SR, Rowley BD: Unethical and unprofessional conduct observed by residents during their first year of training. Acad Med 73:1195–1200, 1998

Bebeau MJ, Thoma SJ: The impact of a dental ethics curriculum on moral reasoning. J Dent Educ 58:684–692, 1994

Bellini LM, Baime M, Shea JA: Variation of mood and empathy during internship. JAMA 287:3143–3146, 2002

Bloch S, Chodoff P, Green SA (eds): Psychiatric Ethics, 3rd Edition. Oxford, UK, Oxford University Press, 1999

Coverdale JH, Bayer T, Isbell P, et al: Are we teaching psychiatrists to be ethical? Acad Psychiatry 16:199–205, 1992

Ende J, Pozen JT, Levinsky NG: Enhancing learning during a clinical clerkship: the value of a structured curriculum. J Gen Intern Med 1:232–237, 1986

Feudtner C, Christakis DA, Christakis NA: Do clinical clerks suffer ethical erosion? Students' perceptions of their ethical environment and personal development. Acad Med 69:670–679, 1994

Firth-Cozens J: Emotional distress in junior house officers. Br Med J (Clin Res Ed) 295:533–536, 1987

Gann PH, Anderson S, Regan MB: Shifts in medical student beliefs about AIDS after a comprehensive training experience. Am J Prev Med 7:172–177, 1991

Green B, Miller PD, Routh CP: Teaching ethics in psychiatry: a one-day workshop for clinical students. J Med Ethics 21:234–238, 1995

Hughes PH, Baldwin DC Jr, Sheehan DV, et al: Resident physician substance use, by specialty. Am J Psychiatry 149:1348–1354, 1992

Jacobson JA, Tolle SW, Stocking C, et al: Internal medicine residents' preferences regarding medical ethics education. Acad Med 64:760–764, 1989

Jex SM, Hughes P, Storr C, et al: Relations among stressors, strains, and substance use among resident physicians. Int J Addict 27:979–994, 1992

Jonsen AR, Siegler M, Winslade WJ: Clinical Ethics, 4th Edition. New York, McGraw-Hill, 1998

Junek W, Burra P, Leichner P: Teaching interviewing skills by encountering patients. J Med Educ 54:402–407, 1979

Junkerman C, Schiedermayer D: Practical Ethics for Students, Interns and Residents. A Short Reference Manual, 2nd Edition. Frederick, MD, University Publishing Group, 1998

Lo B, Schroeder SA: Frequency of ethical dilemmas in a medical inpatient service. Arch Intern Med 141:1062–1064, 1981

Roberts LW, McCarty T, Lyketsos C, et al: What and how psychiatry residents at ten training programs wish to learn ethics. Acad Psychiatry 20:131–143, 1996

Roberts LW, McCarty T, Roberts BB, et al: Clinical ethics teaching in psychiatric supervision. Acad Psychiatry 20:172–184, 1996

Scheidt PC, Lazoritz S, Ebbeling WL, et al: Evaluation of system providing feedback to students on videotaped patient encounters. J Med Educ 61:585–590, 1986

Self DJ, Olivarez M, Baldwin DC Jr: The amount of small-group case-study discussion needed to improve moral reasoning skills of medical students. Acad Med 73:521–523, 1998

Sulmasy DP, Geller G, Levine DM, et al: Medical house officers' knowledge, attitudes, and confidence regarding medical ethics. Arch Intern Med 150:2509–2513, 1990

Sulmasy DP, Terry PB, Faden SR, et al: Long-term effects of ethics education on the quality of care for patients who have do-not-resuscitate orders [see comments]. J Gen Intern Med 9:622–626, 1994

Chapter 16.   Ethical Issues in Psychiatric Research

Advisory Committee on Human Radiation Experiments: The Human Radiation Experiments: Final Report of the President's Advisory Committee. New York, Oxford University Press, 1996

Appelbaum PS, Grisso T: The MacArthur Competence Study I, II, III. Law and Human Behavior 19:105–174, 1995

Appelbaum PS, Roth LH, Lidz C: The therapeutic misconception: informed consent in psychiatric research. Int J Law Psychiatry 5(3–4):319–329, 1982

Beecher HK: Ethics and clinical research. N Engl J Med 274:1354–1360, 1966

Dresser R: Mentally disabled research subjects. The enduring policy issues. JAMA 276:67–72, 1996

Hoagwood K, Jensen PS, Fisher CB (eds): Ethical Issues in Mental Health Research With Children and Adolescents. Mahwah, NJ, Lawrence Erlbaum, 1996

Levine RJ: Ethics and Regulation of Clinical Research. Baltimore, MD, Urban & Schwarzenberg, 1986

National Bioethics Advisory Commission: Research Involving Subjects With Mental Disorders That May Affect Decisionmaking Capacity. Rockville, MD, National Bioethics Advisory Commission, 1998

National Commission for the Protection of Human Subjects of Biomedical and Behavioral Research: The Belmont Report: Ethical Principles and Guidelines for the Protection of Human Subjects of Research. Washington, DC, U.S. Government Printing Office, 1979

Orlans FB, Beauchamp TL, Dresser R, et al: The Human Use of Animals: Case Studies in Ethical Choice. Oxford, UK, Oxford University Press, 1998

Roberts LW: The ethical basis of psychiatric research: conceptual issues and empirical findings. Compr Psychiatry 39:99–110, 1998

Roberts LW: Ethics and mental illness research. Psychiatr Clin North Am 25:525–545, 2002

Roberts LW: Informed consent and the capacity for voluntarism. Am J Psychiatry 159:705–712, 2002

Roberts LW, Geppert CM, Brody JL: A framework for considering the ethical aspects of psychiatric research protocols. Compr Psychiatry 42: 351–363, 2001

Spece RG, Shimm DS, Buchanan AE: Conflicts of Interest in Clinical Practice and Research. New York, Oxford University Press, 1996

Wallerstein N: Power between evaluator and community: research relationships within New Mexico's healthier communities. Soc Sci Med 49:39–53, 1999

Chapter 17.   Health Care Ethics Committees

Ad Hoc Committee of the Harvard Medical School to Examine the Definition of Brain Death: A definition of irreversible coma. JAMA 205:337–340, 1968

Altman LK: Two doctors cited for work developing artificial kidney. New York Times, September 22, 2002

Aulisio MP, Arnold RM, Youngner SJ: Health care ethics consultation: nature, goals, and competencies. A position paper from the Society for Health and Human Values—Society for Bioethics Consultation Task Force on Standards for Bioethics Consultation. Ann Intern Med 133:59–69, 2000

Beecher HK: Ethics and clinical research. N Engl J Med 274:1354–1360, 1966

Drane JF: Clinical Bioethics: Theory and Practice in Medical Ethical Decision-Making. Kansas City, MO, Sheed & Ward, 1994

Fletcher JC, Lombardo PA, Marshall MF, et al. (eds): Introduction to Clinical Ethics, 2nd Edition. Hagerstown, MD, University Publishing Group, 1997

Galla JH: Clinical practice guideline on shared decision-making in the appropriate initiation of and withdrawal from dialysis. Renal Physicians Association and the American Society of Nephrology. J Am Soc Nephrol 11(7):1340–1342, 2000

Katz J: The Nuremberg Code and the Nuremberg Trial. JAMA 276:1662–1666, 1996

Lo B: Behind closed doors: promises and pitfalls of ethics committees. N Engl J Med 317:46–49, 1987

Moreno JD: Consensus, contracts, and committees. Journal of Medicine and Philosophy 16(4):393–408, 1991

National Commission for the Protection of Human Subjects of Biomedical and Behavioral Research: The Belmont Report: Ethical Principles and Guidelines for the Protection of Human Subjects of Research. Washington, DC, U.S. Government Printing Office, 1979

Ross JW: Handbook for Hospital Ethics Committees. Chicago, IL, American Hospital Publishing, 1986

Ross JW, Glaser JM, Rasinski-Gregory D, et al: Health Care Ethics Committees: The Next Generation. Chicago, IL, American Hospital Publishing, 1983

World Medical Association: The Declaration of Helsinki: recommendations guiding medical doctors in biomedical research involving human subjects. JAMA 277:925–926, 1997

INDEX

*Page numbers in **boldface** type refer to tables or figures.*

346

348